T0076640

Guide to the Psychiatry of Old Age

Second edition

Guide to the Psychiatry of Old Age

Second edition

David Ames
University of Melbourne

Damien Gallagher
University of Toronto

Samantha Loi
Royal Melbourne Hospital

Tom Russ
University of Edinburgh & NHS Lothian

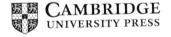
CAMBRIDGE
UNIVERSITY PRESS

CAMBRIDGE
UNIVERSITY PRESS

University Printing House, Cambridge CB2 8BS, United Kingdom

One Liberty Plaza, 20th Floor, New York, NY 10006, USA

477 Williamstown Road, Port Melbourne, VIC 3207, Australia

314–321, 3rd Floor, Plot 3, Splendor Forum, Jasola District Centre,
New Delhi – 110025, India

103 Penang Road, #05–06/07, Visioncrest Commercial, Singapore 238467

Cambridge University Press is part of the University of Cambridge.

It furthers the University's mission by disseminating knowledge in the pursuit of
education, learning, and research at the highest international levels of excellence.

www.cambridge.org
Information on this title: www.cambridge.org/9781108407151
DOI: 10.1017/9781108290173

First edition © D. Ames, E. Chiu, J. Lindesay, K. I. Shulman 2010
Second edition © David Ames, Damien Gallagher, Samantha Loi and Tom Russ 2022

This publication is in copyright. Subject to statutory exception
and to the provisions of relevant collective licensing agreements,
no reproduction of any part may take place without the written
permission of Cambridge University Press.

First published 2010
Reprinted 2012
Second edition 2022

A catalogue record for this publication is available from the British Library.

Library of Congress Cataloging-in-Publication Data
Names: Ames, David, 1954– author. | Gallagher, Damien, author. | Loi, Samantha, author. | Russ, Tom, Dr.
author.
Title: Guide to the psychiatry of old age / David Ames, Damien Gallagher, Samantha Loi, Tom Russ.
Description: 2nd edition. | Cambridge, United Kingdom ; New York, NY : Cambridge University Press,
2022. | Preceded by Guide to the psychiatry of old age / David Ames ... [et al.]. 2010. | Includes
bibliographical references and index.
Identifiers: LCCN 2021036735 (print) | LCCN 2021036736 (ebook) | ISBN 9781108407151 (paperback) |
ISBN 9781108290173 (ebook)
Subjects: MESH: Mental Disorders | Aged | Geriatric Psychiatry – methods
Classification: LCC RC451.4.A5 (print) | LCC RC451.4.A5 (ebook) | NLM WT 150 | DDC 618.97/689–dc23
LC record available at https://lccn.loc.gov/2021036735
LC ebook record available at https://lccn.loc.gov/2021036736

ISBN 978-1-108-40715-1 Paperback

Cambridge University Press has no responsibility for the persistence or accuracy of
URLs for external or third-party internet websites referred to in this publication
and does not guarantee that any content on such websites is, or will remain,
accurate or appropriate.

....

Every effort has been made in preparing this book to provide accurate and up-to-date information that is in
accord with accepted standards and practice at the time of publication. Although case histories are drawn
from actual cases, every effort has been made to disguise the identities of the individuals involved.
Nevertheless, the authors, editors, and publishers can make no warranties that the information contained
herein is totally free from error, not least because clinical standards are constantly changing through research
and regulation. The authors, editors, and publishers therefore disclaim all liability for direct or consequential
damages resulting from the use of material contained in this book. Readers are strongly advised to pay careful
attention to information provided by the manufacturer of any drugs or equipment that they plan to use.

Second edition dedicated to Richard Marley and Roz Seath

Contents

Authors

David Ames
University of Melbourne

Damien Gallagher
University of Toronto

Samantha Loi
Royal Melbourne Hospital

Tom Russ
University of Edinburgh & NHS Lothian

Foreword to the Second Edition

It has been one of the great pleasures of my life to observe and participate in the growth of a specialty which hardly existed when I entered it over 40 years ago. The mental health needs of older people are now much more widely recognised than they were in those early days. Dementia, in particular, has risen up the public agenda with the name of Alzheimer now familiar to everyone. For younger readers, it may be difficult to believe that only 40 years ago this name would have rung no bells even with generally well-informed members of the public.

Growth in knowledge has not stopped over recent years. In the little more than a decade since the first edition of this excellent book was published, new evidence has emerged often to support statements made in the first edition which, at that time, were based more on opinion than on scientific findings. For example, in thinking of primary prevention of dementia, the idea that 'what is good for the heart is also good for the brain' is now well established scientifically. Indeed, some new preventable risk items, such as deafness, have been added to the already substantial list of lifestyle factors, such as a healthy diet, regular exercise and total smoking abstinence, that are relevant to prevention.

The main change since I entered the field, well documented in this book, is in the demographics. The vastly increased expectation of life means that the proportion of older people in countries all over the world, but especially in those that are economically less developed, is much, much greater. In 1970, life expectancy in my country, the United Kingdom, was just under 72; now, in 2021, it is just over 81, a 10-year increase. There have also been highly relevant changes in family structure. Increases in the divorce rate mean that there is now far more social isolation and loneliness in the older population with implications for rates of depression and how it needs to be managed.

These demographic changes carry important implications, well described here, for all health professionals dealing with older people, and these are by no means limited to those working in specialist services. Those working in primary care, whether as doctors or nurses or in other para-medical professions need to have a sound knowledge of the variety of mental health problems in older people, how to recognise them, assess them and deal with them. So far, the training of non-specialist health professionals, even in economically developed countries, has been inadequate in this respect. For example, the fact that frail older people are more often than not suffering from *both* physical *and* mental health problems is so little recognised that often one or the other is ignored. The lesson I learned from my first mentor in the field, Professor Tom Arie, recently sadly deceased, is that family practitioners, geriatricians and old age psychiatrists need to train and work together has still not been fully appreciated. This book is an invaluable resource for students and those responsible for such training, not only in economically developed but also in economically less developed countries.

The need for such knowledge is not confined to those working in health settings. It is now widely understood that many of the people receiving residential and social care often have dementia and other mental health problems like depression. Training of all staff working in these facilities requires understanding of the way mental health problems such as dementia develop over time, from the first indications of mild memory loss through to severe cognitive impairment with its implications extending right through to end-of-life care. The need to train those working in social care as well as to improve their status by giving them better pay and career prospects is clear. Again, those engaged in such training will find this book helpful in planning their courses.

Finally, a word about the future. The authors of this book, while not neglecting other approaches, in their discussion of likely future developments, give main prominence to the neurosciences and genetics. It is certainly the case that this is where research resources and efforts have been and are currently concentrated. My own view is that, despite the vast amount of neuroscience research over the last 40 years, with fascinating findings, the amount of *clinical* impact of this new knowledge has been rather disappointing. I suspect that, in the future, it will be the importance of multidisciplinary work and the nature of the relationship between older people, their family members and the health and social care professionals looking after them that will be seen as of even greater relevance to the quality of their care. Not surprisingly, given my own involvement in it, I would also expect the voluntary sector to assume a higher profile in service provision. But in whichever ways the future develops, this book will remain an invaluable resource.

Nori Graham

Foreword to the First Edition

By the time I launched the first dementia programme at Johns Hopkins in 1979, the psychiatry of old age was well established in the UK. Two small gems from those early days of geriatric psychiatry in the UK – the sections on old age psychiatry in *Clinical Psychiatry* by Mayer-Gross, Slater and Roth and the monograph by Felix Post, *Clinical Psychiatry of Late Life* – influenced my decision to pursue a career in the psychiatry of old age.

This new, brief guide makes geriatric psychiatry accessible to generalists, clinicians not medically trained and even patients and families. Such efforts are needed in these days of ageing populations and shrinking resources to persuade doctors and the public to reject the prejudice of ageism, and to teach that clinical signs and symptoms of elderly patients are the products of diseases and vulnerabilities, just as they are in younger people, and not the inevitable consequences of ageing, which require the discovery of the fountain of youth before the ills of the elderly can be prevented and cured.

In addition to the recognition and explanation of pathological processes causing signs and symptoms, this book promotes the narrative, or meaningful, approach, which illuminates the dignity and right to life of the elderly. The privilege of sharing the stories of almost completed lives is one of the rewards of geriatric practice. In an attempt to demonstrate this to a class of medical students, I interviewed a distinguished 90-year-old American psychiatrist, Mandel Cohen. I expected him to describe the changes he experienced as he grew older. I asked, 'Doctor, what is it like to be old?' He replied, 'I don't feel old in my mind', and he wasn't. Another story that illustrates the dignity of older people and their right to life emerged on an Alzheimer's disease (AD) unit in a nursing home. The question arose as to the validity of documents signed by family members requesting that patients not be resuscitated. In order to answer this question, I gathered a group of 10 severely impaired residents, none of whom had a Mini-mental State Examination (MMSE) score greater than 10 out of 30, and asked them if they wanted to be resuscitated. When one said, 'What does "resuscitated" mean?', another member of the group said, 'You know, brought back to life'. The first person responded, 'Well, you have to make allowances for people with memory trouble'. Seven of 10 said they wanted resuscitation. The ones who didn't appeared to be depressed. Too often, we fail to honour the dignity of cognitively impaired elderly by asking them if they want to live, and if they don't want to live by giving them the benefit of an examination to determine if their decision was the product of a pathological process causing dementia or depression. I would highlight a few aspects of the contemporary assessment, diagnosis and treatment of psychiatric disorders of the elderly surveyed by this book. The first is the importance of using a quantitative cognitive examination for clinical decision-making and for educating patients and families. Although cognitive examinations can be performed by specialists such as neuropsychologists, the treating clinician should examine the patient and be able to explain the results in appropriate terms to the patient and family. The important point here is not which of the several available tests is used, but that clinicians should use some quantitative method suitable for the clinical situation and purpose. Just as medicine was advanced by the introduction of the thermometer, psychiatry has been advanced by the introduction of quantitative methods of assessment. Before the modern thermometer was introduced 150 years ago, physicians felt the skin temperature and judged whether it was too warm. This method was good enough to appreciate the importance of fever, but it was not good enough to measure reliably whether the temperature was rising or falling. Today, it is not enough for the clinician to say that a patient is confused when it is possible to describe quantitatively the severity of the various impairments and to determine by serial measurement whether impairments are improving or worsening.

The second issue I would like to emphasize is the authors' discussion of that murky diagnostic category, pseudodementia. This term was usually intended to mean that a patient's cognitive impairment was not due to a neuropathological abnormality, and it implied that all true dementias were irreversible. Pseudodementia was usually applied to elderly persons with depression and cognitive impairment. Follow-up studies indicate that many of the patients so labelled do deteriorate and some have AD. This kind of evidence has been influential in returning the term dementia to its intended usage: deterioration of multiple cognitive functions in clear consciousness, without specifying either aetiology or reversibility. Instead of pseudodementia, designations such as 'depression with cognitive impairment' or 'dementia of depression' are better descriptors of the condition. This usage also encourages the point of view that depression in the elderly, both in the presence and absence of AD, should be a focus of treatment.

Finally, I would like to draw attention to the authors' discussion of currently used medications and their side effects. In some circumstances, 'reverse pharmacology' – stopping many if not all medications – leads to cognitive improvement. In other circumstances, doctors recommend medications even though treatment options are limited, because there are no curative drugs and the available symptomatic remedies carry substantial risk. In this unhappy situation, the doctors must explain the options to the patient and family and encourage them to collaborate in the decision as to whether the benefits are greater than the risks. This discussion is useful because it offers hope that something can be done or at least that no harm will be done, and it conveys to the patient and family the physicians' respect for cognitively impaired people, who often perceive that their clinicians do not consider them worthy of their efforts.

This brief guide is a welcome addition to the distinguished publications about geriatric psychiatry from the UK and more recently from many other countries. In addition to introducing the field to students and generalists, this brief book might even persuade some young student to join the field, just as 40 years ago one small book and a small part of a larger book written by their predecessors steered me into a satisfying career, which gave me the opportunity to teach, to learn from and to collaborate with many elderly patients and their families in order to enable them to choose to live as best they could, given their individual circumstances.

Marshal Folstein

Preface to the Second Edition

In 2014 the late Richard Marley suggested to David Ames that a second edition of this text should be prepared. Three of the four original authors, having progressed to various stages of retirement, graciously consented to forego authorship and for the text of the first edition to form a basis for a second edition to be revised and rewritten by a new team led by Ames. We thank them for their excellent work on the first edition and for opening an opportunity for three younger colleagues to become authors. Thus, three new collaborators from Toronto, Melbourne and Edinburgh, together with Ames, set about the work of updating and improving the text and recommended reading for each of the original 12 chapters. The eminent psychiatrist Professor Marshal Folstein, famous for developing the Mini-mental State Examination, was kind enough to write a generous foreword for the first edition; we were fortunate in being able to persuade Dr Nori Graham to provide one for this second edition. Nori Graham oversaw the initiation of, and then ran, psychiatric services for older people in the London borough of Camden for many years, facilitating the training of a large number of old age psychiatrists, nurses and allied health staff, and running a model service for older people with dementia and functional psychiatric disorders. She mentored Ames in both clinical work and his doctoral research and was a highly influential president of Alzheimer's Disease International during a long career devoted to helping those with psychiatric disorders in late life, and their carers. We thank her for taking the time out of a still busy schedule to write the foreword for this book.

Any tardiness in the production of this volume is entirely due to dilatoriness and distraction on the part of Ames, himself now close to retirement as well (the title of Emeritus Professor having been conferred in 2016 can be decoded as 'E' means you're out and 'meritus' means you deserve to be; these lines were uttered by Barry Humphries playing the part of Rupert Murdoch in the TV show *The Hitler Diaries*). However, delay is not always a bad thing. The 11 years between the release of the first edition to the submission of the text for the second have seen a number of new developments in the psychiatry of old age; many of these are reflected in this updated version of the book. All chapters have been revised, their reading lists enhanced with more recent publications, and one of them has been rewritten from scratch.

We hope that a new generation of medical students, trainee psychiatrists, general practitioners and geriatricians, nurses and allied health professionals, from a multitude of countries, will find this second edition as useful as some of their predecessors have told us they found the first one.

Our thanks are due to the patient staff at Cambridge University Press, whose gentle encouragement kept the show on the road when it looked like grinding to a halt or veering into a ditch. This edition is dedicated to Richard Marley, a superb editor, generous colleague and good friend, taken before his time, but not forgotten by those of us who had the privilege to work with him, and to Roz Seath, secretary extraordinaire to Ed Chiu, David Ames and their colleague Nicola Lautenschlager, whose dedication to her role was reflected in the high regard she was held by many international and Australian colleagues who came to know her through her work with three professors of old age psychiatry over more than three decades.

David Ames, Damien Gallagher, Samantha Loi and Tom Russ

Preface to the First Edition

With rapid ageing of the world population, the psychiatry of old age (POA) has become a crucial discipline, because rates of dementia, delirium and late life functional psychiatric disorders, such as depression, are increasing quickly in both the developed and developing world as a consequence of the sustained and unprecedented increase in the number of older people. In many developed countries the subspecialty of psychiatry of old age (also known as old age psychiatry, psychogeriatrics, geriatric psychiatry, geropsychiatry) is now well established, with over 500 subspecialists in the UK and 200 in Australia. Special training programmes for the discipline have been operating in several countries for some years now, and often completion of these programmes leads to the award of a certificate of competence in the psychiatry of old age. In developing countries, especially those with rising affluence, there is emerging interest in the subspecialty and recognition of the need for service providers to acquire expertise in the area. In addition, most basic training programmes for general psychiatrists now require some exposure to and knowledge of POA, and we hope that this trend will strengthen as old people approach one quarter of the total population in many places.

Despite this need, although there are excellent comprehensive, detailed and expensive texts on POA, there are fewer good, short, inexpensive books on this subject, and those that exist tend to have a national rather than an international focus.

For this reason, supported by Cambridge University Press and with the endorsement of the International Psychogeriatric Association (IPA), the four of us resolved to write a book on POA that would be short, comprehensive and affordable. In making this decision we were mindful of both an apparent unmet need and the involvement that all four of us have had with IPA over many years (all of us have been members of IPA's Board of Directors, Edmond Chiu was IPA secretary and then president and Ames has edited IPA's peer reviewed journal *International Psychogeriatrics* since 2003). This, after a prolonged gestation and writing process, is the result. It is aimed at trainee psychiatrists, higher trainees in the psychiatry of old age, geriatricians and trainee geriatricians, general psychiatrists, neurologists, physicians in training, general practitioners, allied health staff, nurses and medical students. We hope that our audience will be international, so the book's content is not limited solely to the experiences of POA in the three countries in which the authors have lived and worked, but is informed by our experiences of visiting, teaching and talking to our colleagues in a wide variety of countries around the world.

In order to keep the book at a relatively manageable size, the text is not referenced with citations for every statement made, but we hope that the suggestions for further reading given at the end of each chapter (many of which are available free of charge to members of IPA) will be found to be up to date and helpful by our readers.

We trust that health practitioners around the world will find this to be a useful book and that in due course a second edition will be needed. To that end we encourage readers to suggest to us how this edition could be improved.

Books like this do not appear without the help and assistance of a large number of people. We are grateful to Richard Marley and his colleagues at Cambridge University Press (Cambridge University Press is an IPA corporate partner and has published *International*

Psychogeriatrics, IPA's peer-reviewed journal, since 2004) for their encouragement to write the book and their patience when the first author's numerous other responsibilities slowed down its creation. Nisha Doshi has worked tirelessly to refine the copy that was submitted into the elegant text that you now hold. Susan Oster, the executive director of IPA, was consistently enthusiastic about this project, especially the idea of offering copies to IPA members at discounted cost. Leonardo Pantoni (IPA publications committee chair) and Michael Philpot (book review editor of *International Psychogeriatrics*) checked the text rapidly at short notice to ensure that its content was compatible with IPA's mission and values, and we are very grateful to them for doing this so quickly and cheerfully, and for their many useful and thoughtful suggestions which improved the final text. Roz Seath gave tireless and invaluable secretarial support to this project, as she has done for more books than we, or she, would care to count. The book was completed during the last three months of 2009 when Ames was on sabbatical leave from his research institute and university – the hospitality and kindness of Craig Ritchie and his Imperial College colleagues at Charing Cross Hospital, London, during this time helped to make possible the book's completion. Finally, we would like to thank our patients and their families – from them we have learned most of what little we know about this expanding and intriguing branch of medicine.

David Ames, Edmond Chiu, James Lindesay and Ken Shulman

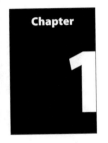

Chapter

1

What Is the Psychiatry of Old Age and Why Do We Need It?

The psychiatry of old age (POA) is concerned with the identification, assessment, treatment and care of older adults with mental disorders, and of those who care for them. Mental illness in late life is as old as humanity, and there is a long history of social and medical interventions with affected individuals, some more enlightened than others. Traditionally, the care of older people has been centred in the family, and it is only when this source of support is absent or insufficient that the local community or the State has intervened. In mediaeval Europe, the legislation developed for this purpose had as much to do with the management of property as the welfare of the individual, but the records show that in the context of small and relatively cohesive communities, it could deliver sophisticated and effective care for insane and incompetent individuals, both rich and poor. The modern history of old age psychiatry in developed societies has its origins in the changing social demography of the nineteenth century, with the rapid urbanisation of populations and growth in the numbers of old people. With local community support no longer sustainable, the poor and the disabled (older people were often both) were particularly vulnerable. The responses to this welfare challenge were many and various, and included poor laws, pensions and institutional solutions such as workhouses, infirmaries and lunatic asylums. Within these institutions, often later re-labelled as 'hospitals', the frailties of old age were medicalised, and became the professional responsibility of physicians and psychiatrists. So far as mental illness was concerned, however, this was not a responsibility that was especially welcomed by anyone. Mental illnesses in older adults were believed to be degenerative or 'senile' and thus not amenable to treatment. There was particular therapeutic nihilism regarding people with dementia; they could not be discharged from acute medical beds, psychiatrists were not equipped to deal with the problem and no one had anything to offer beyond institutional warehousing in nursing homes or the chronic wards of the old asylums.

This professional pessimism and lack of interest began to be challenged in the second half of the twentieth century by small groups of innovators, particularly in the United Kingdom. The creation of 'geriatric medicine' within the National Health Service (NHS, established 1948), with its avowed interest in all of the physical and mental problems of older people, and its multi-professional approach to solving them, was an important model for the later development of old age psychiatry by pioneers such as Tom Arie and Tony Whitehead. An important factor influencing this change of attitude in service providers was research. In 1944, Martin (later Sir Martin) Roth in the United Kingdom established the modern nosology of what was originally thought to be a single degenerative illness, demonstrating that not all mental illness in old age has the same bad prognosis, and that mortality in individuals with affective and psychotic disorders was much less than in those with dementia. This optimism was encouraged by the successful application of both physical and social treatments to older patients. A number of large epidemiological studies of mental disorders in community populations aged over 60 or 65 were carried out at this time in the United States, Scandinavia and the United Kingdom, which characterised the full range of these conditions (especially dementia, depression and schizophrenia-like disorders), and the extent to which those affected by them were out of touch with any services. These surveys showed that only a minority of the elderly population was mentally ill; an important message from the emerging science of gerontology was that physical and mental frailty was by no means the inevitable consequence of ageing, and that the compression of morbidity was a realistic and achievable goal.

Another important factor driving change in service provision for older people in high-income countries has been government health policy, developed in response to demographic ageing, the cost-effectiveness of treatment and care and rising expectations of people regarding the quality of that care. By the 1960s, it was widely accepted that the traditional custodial approach to the care of the mentally ill was no longer acceptable, and that the focus of services should move to the home and the community. However, the rate and extent of the development of community-based old age psychiatry services have differed substantially between countries: those with universal health and social care funding and centralised health policy and planning, such as the United Kingdom and Canada, have created much more comprehensive services than those without universal coverage. Active and vocal voluntary and other non-government organisations, such as the Alzheimer's Association (United States), Alzheimer's Society and Alzheimer's Scotland (United Kingdom), Dementia Australia and Alzheimer's Disease International (ADI), have been a valuable stimulus to service development, particularly for the support of carers. The development of services for older adults with mental illness, and the international consensus model of their organisation published by the World Psychiatric Association in 1997, are discussed in detail in Chapter 11.

The Future

Developed societies were the first to experience demographic ageing and the growth in the number of older people with mental illness, but the rest of the world is catching up fast. The World Health Organisation (WHO) estimated that in 2020 there were about 50 million people with dementia in the world, with 10 million new cases annually. The number of those affected by dementia is projected to increase to 152 million by 2050. Most people with dementia live in low- and middle-income countries.

Dementia is not the only disorder that will increase in prevalence with demographic ageing. Other conditions, such as vascular disease, arthritis and sensory impairments, will contribute to an increasing burden of chronic physical and mental disability in old age, as will emerging problems such as the global epidemic of obesity. Other factors will have an impact upon the future welfare and care of older people too. For example, in developed societies, the shifting dependency ratio of the population will require individuals to continue working beyond traditional retirement age, as they always have done in poorer countries. Increased geographic mobility, with children moving away from home and parents relocating on retirement, will reduce the availability of informal care, as will the continued growth in the number of single-person households. Changing cultural ideals, such as Confucianism or collectivism with migration and increased 'Westernisation', also may contribute to the care of older and frail adults being left to the State, rather than the family. In the developing world, there will be the challenge of competing demands of young and old for healthcare, particularly for conditions, such as Acquired Immune Deficiency Syndrome (AIDS), that disproportionately affect younger, economically active age groups. For some countries, rapid economic growth may help to some extent with the challenges of demographic ageing, but this will bring complications as well, such as the economic migration of younger people into cities and to more affluent countries. In many places, the stigma associated with mental disorder at all ages is a major obstacle to care provision. There are other, less predictable, eventualities that could have a major impact upon the capacity of all societies to respond to demographic ageing in the years to come, for example the COVID-19 pandemic, which has led to disproportionate mortality among the very old and frail and has caused major social and economic disruption, or climate change bringing about damage to infrastructure, large-scale population movements and potential resource wars. On a more positive note, there would be considerable economic and social benefits globally were we to achieve effective control of widespread endemic diseases such as malaria at last.

These projections and predictions have profound social and economic implications for both developed and developing societies around the world. Even the richest nations may struggle to maintain levels of health and social care at their current levels, and for much of the developing world the models of service infrastructure pioneered in the United Kingdom and other developed countries simply are not suitable or practical. In the likely absence of cheap and simple cures for disorders, such as dementia, other approaches will have to be found. This has led to a greater public health focus on primary prevention, particularly the prevention of cerebrovascular disease through effective control of vascular risk factors such as hypertension, diabetes and smoking. The quest to develop 'disease-modifying therapies' that may prevent or delay the progression of Alzheimer's disease (AD) continues, but such treatments may only be effective if used in the preclinical stages of the disease, before neuropathological damage has reached a critical point. There is also a body of evidence to indicate that the onset of clinical dementia may be delayed in individuals with a greater 'cognitive reserve', suggesting that improved nutrition and education in childhood and young adulthood may have a positive effect on the incidence of dementia in late life. Research continues on strategies to boost cognitive reserve; the 'use it or lose it' hypothesis is attractive, but the evidence is still evolving and the evidence from studies assessing the impact of exercise, social engagement and cognitive stimulation in late life report, at best, only small effect sizes for the benefit to cognition. So far as secondary prevention is concerned, there will be a need to develop new service models for societies that can afford only basic levels of healthcare. Inevitably, these will need to build upon what already exists, for example by developing and extending the role of those professionals, such as nurses, who currently visit families at home. The focus of their new role would be upon improved detection and increasing carer support, through information, training and development of local community solutions where possible. Public education will be critical to increase understanding of mental illness in late life, and to combat the associated stigma.

Further Reading

Articles

Livingston, G. *et al.* (2020). Dementia prevention, intervention, and care: 2020 report of the Lancet Commission. *Lancet,* 396, 413–446. doi: 10.1016/S0140-6736(20)30367-6.

Comprehensive review and summary of the literature, including evidence for prevention of dementia, compiled and revised in 2018–2019.

Wertheimer, J. (1997). Psychiatry of the elderly: a consensus statement. *International Journal of Geriatric Psychiatry*, 12, 432–435. doi: 10.1002/(sici)1099-1166(199704)12:4<432:: aid-gps1576>3.0.co;2-s.

The principles outlined in this editorial remain highly relevant today.

Website

www.who.int/news-room/fact-sheets/detail/ dementia Access 31st January 2021.

A source for up-to-date facts about the global prevalence, incidence and impact of dementia.

Book

Dening, T. and Thomas, A. (eds.). (2020). *Oxford Textbook of Old Age Psychiatry*, 3rd ed., Oxford: Oxford University Press.

Easily the best comprehensive multi-author textbook on the subspecialty.

Psychiatric Assessment of Older Adults

Introduction

The assessment of older adults with psychiatric or cognitive symptoms requires a broad range of knowledge and skills. Hence, the psychiatry of old age (POA) has been referred to as 'general psychiatry only more so'! This chapter outlines the special features that characterise the assessment of older adults with psychiatric symptoms. In particular, we focus upon the additional skills necessary to complete a comprehensive psychiatric assessment in older, compared to younger, adults. These skills include: (1) increased flexibility regarding the place and mode of assessment; (2) incorporating information provided by an informant or carer as an essential aspect of the assessment; (3) understanding the trajectory of mental health disorders throughout life; (4) understanding medical comorbidity, especially of neurological disorders and the impact of commonly used medications; (5) being able to complete a cognitive assessment, including frontal and executive processes commonly implicated in neuropsychiatric disorders.

Where to Assess the Patient

The doctor's office is an appropriate setting for most patients who are high functioning, cooperative and competent. However, this is not the case for many older adults who may have significant cognitive impairment, mobility difficulties and frailty. In such instances, the patient's own home setting is preferred. This approach is often necessary and allows for more accurate assessment of the impact of environmental factors, safety issues and daily functioning in the home environment.

In older adults, the complex and multifaceted nature of clinical presentations invites the involvement of other healthcare professionals to address psychosocial issues and other environmental factors of practical concern. Ideally, the psychiatrist is part of a multidisciplinary team that can address medical, cognitive, behavioural and psychological issues while attending to practical concerns such as safety, nutrition, mobility and the well-being of carers. A multidisciplinary team based in or closely affiliated with a hospital may more readily have access to medical consultations and investigations. Because of the high prevalence of medical comorbidity, access to these resources is essential. One may need to rule out common conditions such as ischaemic heart disease, heart failure, hypothyroidism, vitamin deficiencies, hepatic and renal dysfunction or electrolyte imbalances. Hence, ready access to laboratory services is necessary. Neuroimaging is needed for the assessment of neurocognitive disorders. In particular, access to neuroimaging is required either to rule in or rule out common causes of neuropsychiatric disorders and to assess for potentially reversible causes of cognitive decline.

Because of the high frequency of medical comorbidity and prescribed medications, it is advisable that all psychiatric assessments of older adults involve the patient's general practitioner (GP/primary care physician) and other healthcare professionals contributing to the patient's care. The initial assessment is typically conducted by the GP who may then refer to a POA service where the diagnosis is unclear or management considerations are complex.

Involving the Carer and/or Informant

In the past, and particularly in younger adults, concerns regarding confidentiality and the primacy of the doctor–patient relationship may have resulted in carers or other key family members being excluded from the assessment and management of major psychiatric disorders. This is typically not the case for older adults where, because of physical infirmity or cognitive decline, carers and family members are often more intimately involved in the patient's care. In fact, obtaining a collateral history from a family member or carer is an integral part of the assessment process for older adults. The absence of a carer or informant limits the quality and accuracy of the information obtained and impacts negatively upon the patient's care. Therefore, we suggest that, where possible, all psychiatric assessments of older adults should include an informant or carer who has a good understanding of the patient's functioning and behaviour. Carers and family members are often considered equal partners in the therapeutic alliance that develops with the psychiatrist and the multidiscip-linary healthcare team. The traditional dyad of 'doctor/patient relationship' is often trans-formed into the 'doctor/family relationship' in POA. This must be the case when the patient is incapable, cognitively impaired or extremely frail and vulnerable. In this situation the carer is often acting in the capacity of an enduring power of attorney for personal care or under the authority of an advanced healthcare directive.

Whether one should interview the patient or carer first or both together is an important consideration and may be determined by the clinical circumstances. It is often helpful to elicit the reason for presentation both from the patient and carer perspectives initially, which will then help guide the interview format. In circumstances where the patient is cognitively impaired and apparently has few concerns because they have limited insight, the focus of the interview will necessarily be with the carer or family member. This is particu-larly true for elements in the history relating to daily functioning and safety, regarding which the patient may have limited awareness. Of course, the quality of collateral informa-tion provided will depend upon the informant's frequency of contact with the patient and the informant's own state of health and health literacy. It is critical to ensure that the carer best positioned to provide accurate collateral information is seen with the patient for both assessment and review visits.

If the patient and family member are seen together, this may inhibit the latter's ability to provide a full and honest history. In such circumstances, a family member may censor their history because they do not wish to offend the patient or may fear the consequences of speaking openly. This may be avoided by interviewing the carer separately. Similarly, in circumstances where there are concerns regarding exploitation or abuse of a vulnerable person, it is critical to interview the patient separately and, where necessary, obtain further collateral information from other carers or family members. Cognitive testing can be compromised by a well-meaning family member trying to 'help' the patient. If the patient is anxious, because of others present in the room, this may limit their attention and engagement with cognitive testing. Conversely, useful information can be gleaned from observing the interactions between the patient and carer together, which sometimes can be problematic and may influence care recommendations. Having completed the assessment and established a management plan, it is usually best to see the patient and family together to minimise divergent interpretations of the assessment and management plan.

Carer Perceptions

As a general rule, carers are usually accurate when they indicate that there has been a change in the patient's behaviour or level of functioning. However, their interpretation of why the behaviour has changed may be inaccurate. For example, carers may misinterpret apathy secondary to an evolving neurocognitive disorder as depression or may attribute changes to long-standing personality traits. Carers may feel that the patient is being deliberately obstinate or hostile because of historical interpersonal conflicts. These attributions should be corrected, and it is best to do this at the time of initial assessment.

History Taking

In the vast majority of cases, history taking is the most important element to help establish a provisional diagnosis. The challenge in taking a history from an older adult is that one can be overwhelmed by the many details of a long and eventful life. The clinician should have the capacity to filter relevant from irrelevant information and focus on major events and patterns of behaviour in order to complete the assessment in a timely fashion. It is useful to take a lifespan approach, mindful of the fact that early developmental abnormalities and psychosocial influences can impact upon presentation of psychopathology in later life. It is useful to understand early neurodevelopment and whether there were any major disruptions such as early losses of a parent from death or divorce or significant trauma in childhood. The objective is to obtain an overview of the patterns of adjustment to early relationships, school and work history through to bereavement and health difficulties later on. These facts may then be synthesised into a concise and coherent history with particular focus upon predisposing, precipitating and perpetuating factors that are likely to be relevant to clinical management.

In older adults it is always important to clarify the age of onset of reported psychiatric symptoms or disorders. This provides a clue as to the likely contribution of familial or genetic factors versus acquired degenerative or cerebrovascular changes, which often arise for the first time in later life. For example, depression with first onset in later life is more likely to be associated with neurocognitive decline and less likely to be associated with a positive family history, although clearly environmental influences and predisposing genetic factors are still relevant. Older adults may have acquired coping skills and proven resilient in the face of several adversities throughout their lifetime, raising the question, 'Why now?', when an older adult presents to a psychiatrist for the first time. The answer to this question must be carefully considered as behavioural changes arising for the first time in later life often herald the onset of a neurodegenerative disorder.

In POA it is especially important to have a good understanding of how common medical conditions and their treatments interact with psychiatric disorders. The clinical history should pay close attention to medical comorbidities, their time course and relationship to presenting psychiatric complaints. Furthermore, a detailed review of current medications and recent changes is important when determining whether treatments could have contributed to presenting symptoms. A sound awareness of changing pharmacodynamic and pharmacokinetic considerations in ageing adults and potential interactions between medications is critical for safe prescribing. It is for this reason that the physician-assessor often plays a central role in the initial assessment of older adults referred to a 'POA service'.

Mental State Examination

The mental state examination takes the form of a semi-structured interview and occurs throughout the history-taking process. As in younger adults, the mental state examination begins from the moment one first observes the patient through to the completion of the assessment. Even over the distance from the waiting area to the office, the doctor can complete a preliminary assessment of gait to detect evidence of underlying Parkinsonism or cerebrovascular pathology. What most distinguishes the assessment of older compared to younger adults is the need to do a careful cognitive assessment in all cases. One should resist the inclination to avoid a formal cognitive screen when the patient appears to be superficially intact, as emerging cognitive deficits may be apparent only on testing. This is especially important in individuals who maintain their social graces or may have a high pre-morbid level of functioning that allows them to compensate in ways that may not make their cognitive deficits immediately apparent.

> **Clinical Pearl: Cognitive Screening during the Interview**
>
> It is often helpful informally to assess a patient's cognitive abilities and medical understanding during the clinical interview. Patients with early memory loss or recent episodes of delirium may have an incomplete recollection of recent medical events. It is useful to compare the patient's recollection of events to that documented in their medical records. It is often helpful to check whether they can recall a list of their current medications, as failure to do so should increase suspicion of likely non-adherence.

As is usual in younger adults, it is best to initiate the interview with open-ended questions. Open-ended questions allow the patient to present the issues of primary concern to them, which may then be further explored and addressed during the clinical interview. Failure to allow the patient sufficient time to present their concerns, even when these concerns are peripheral to the primary reason for referral, increases risk of poor therapeutic rapport, dissatisfaction and subsequent non-adherence to treatment recommendations. In addition, the patient's responses to initial open-ended questions may uncover underlying thought disorder, expressive language difficulties or incoherent reasoning, indicative of underlying cognitive dysfunction. Having invested this time at the start of the interview, one may then move towards closed and specific questions, particularly where cognitive impairment or over-inclusiveness preclude more open questioning.

The assessment of appearance, behaviour, speech, thought form and content should proceed in the same way as it would in a younger adult. Self-care and nutritional status are of particular relevance in older adults who may live alone or are in vulnerable circumstances.

Subtle word-finding difficulties, circumlocutions or receptive language difficulties may be evident early on. It is also worth noting that older adults may be less likely to report low mood and may instead present with somatic symptoms when depressed. In the context of memory loss, assessment of mood will require more input from the caregiver. If there is apathy, one should determine whether the apathy is part of a depressive syndrome or secondary to an incipient neurodegenerative condition. In the latter, patients generally present themselves as content, with few or no depressive ruminations, and there is an apparent lack of psychological distress. The cognitive assessment is necessarily more detailed than would be the case in a younger adult because of the high prevalence of cognitive disorders in this age group. This is described in the next section.

Clinical Pearl: The White Roots Sign

Felix Post, one of the original pioneers in POA, has previously referred to the 'white roots sign'. Decline in personal grooming often reflects diminished motivation in the context of a depressive disorder. When an older adult who usually dyes their hair presents with white roots, this may provide an immediate clue. Given that hair grows at the rate of approximately half an inch a month, a two-inch band of white roots may indicate a four-month history of depression! This clinical observation is of course provisional and would need to be corroborated by history and the remainder of the mental state examination. It is also important to differentiate apathy secondary to neurocognitive decline from depression in older adults.

Cognitive Assessment

Cognitive assessment is an essential part of the assessment of older adults. No matter how intact an older adult appears or how preserved the social graces, a formal cognitive assessment is vital. This assessment requires time and patience; older adults are more likely to become fatigued and to have sensory impairments. These sensory impairments should be optimised prior to the assessment, and in some instances, it may be necessary to conduct a full assessment over more than one visit. The cognitive assessment must always be interpreted in the context of the patient's age, educational level and cultural and linguistic background, as performance on cognitive tests is frequently affected by these factors. Many commonly used tests have normative population data available which indicate expected scores for a given age and education. Tests of individual cognitive domains, such as language or memory, theoretically map onto specific neural circuits, although in effect most tests depend upon several functionally integrated neural circuits. Nonetheless, the pattern and progression of cognitive loss can provide some indication as to the underlying neuropathology. The profile on cognitive testing is then integrated with information from the clinical history and with neuroimaging findings to increase diagnostic accuracy. The nature and severity of cognitive deficits will also help determine necessary care supports and care planning. Repeated testing over time can help differentiate cognitive decline from natural progression of disease or detect sudden large changes in cognitive performance such as those that occur in delirium. Whichever cognitive test is used, it is important to administer it in exactly the same way each time to each patient, in order to increase reliability and accuracy of testing.

> **Clinical Pearl: Head Turning Sign**
>
> The 'heard turning sign' is frequently evident in older adults with memory loss. This refers to the patient's tendency to look towards their carer when asked a direct question which depends upon intact short-term memory. The older adult with memory loss may defer to their carer's recollection of recent events and turn expectantly towards them for help when asked a question. This sign, of course, depends on some measure of insight in the patient, which is not always the case.

Which Cognitive Test to Use?

There is a broad range of cognitive tests from which to choose. However, an International Psychogeriatric Association (IPA) survey of brief cognitive screening instruments revealed that geriatric specialists worldwide use a relatively small number of screening instruments. In decreasing order of frequency these included the following instruments: all forms of the Mini-mental State Examination (MMSE; 100%); the Clock-Drawing Test (CDT; 72%); Delayed Recall (56%); Verbal Fluency (39%); Similarities (27%); and the Trail Making Test (25%). Since then the Montreal Cognitive Assessment (MoCA) has entered common usage. The MoCA is more sensitive to mild cognitive impairment (MCI) than the MMSE and several language versions are available. Online training in the administration of the MoCA is available and potential users must undertake this before attempting to utilise the instrument. Recently, the Free-Cog, which integrates measurement of cognition and executive abilities, has shown promise in initial evaluation. Other brief batteries, such as the Mini-Cog and the General Practitioner Assessment of Cognition (GPCOG), combine a short memory test with the CDT and are intended to be used for screening in primary care/general practice. More extensive batteries, including the Addenbrooke's Cognitive Examination (ACE), Cambridge Cognitive Examination (CAMCOG), Neuropsychiatry Unit Cognitive Assessment tool (NUCOG) and the Alzheimer's Disease Assessment Scale, cognitive subscale (ADAS-Cog), take longer to administer but may be more sensitive to change over time. The Rowland Universal Dementia Assessment Scale (RUDAS) was designed to minimise bias secondary to cultural or language variability. In this test the patient is encouraged to communicate in the language in which they are most competent via an interpreter. In summary, there is a broad range of tests from which to choose. An experienced clinician may draw upon a range of tests depending on the clinical context and the purpose of testing. We have summarised certain strengths and weaknesses of commonly used cognitive tests later. This list is not exhaustive and is intended as a brief introduction.

The Mini-mental State Examination

This is the most widely used cognitive screening instrument in the world. The MMSE was developed by Folstein *et al.* in 1975. It is a brief measure of cognitive functioning and takes ≤10 minutes to administer. Despite its limitations, including bias by education, culture and language, and lack of any tests of frontal function, it is still a very useful test. Variants of the MMSE have been developed, including the Standardised Mini-mental State Examination (SMMSE) and the Modified Mini-mental State Examination (MMMSE). It is divided into sections which assess orientation, registration, attention and calculation, recall and language with a maximum score of 30 and an approximate cut-off score of 24 to detect likely dementia depending on age, education and language. It is heavily weighted towards tests of orientation, short-term memory and language with only one visuospatial test (intersecting pentagons). It is important to note that the MMSE does not formally test frontal lobe or executive functions. Frequently, these domains are impaired in neuropsychiatric disorders and if the MMSE is used, additional tests to assess these domains should be added. The MMSE lacks sensitivity in MCI. In addition, this test is subject to copyright, and this fact, in combination with its psychometric limitations, has led to a decrease in its popularity in recent years.

The Clock-Drawing Test

One very popular screening test is the CDT. This test generally uses a pre-drawn circle (approximately 10 cm in diameter) which is placed before the patient with the following instruction: 'This is a clock face. Please fill in the numbers and then set the time to ten past eleven.' One should avoid the use of the word 'hands' as this clue may mask impairment of higher-level functions such as abstract thinking. The CDT has proven to be useful because of the wide range of intellectual functions it subsumes. It casts a wide net that includes functions such as comprehension, planning, visual memory, visuospatial ability, abstract thinking, concentration and motivation. The task of setting the time to ten past eleven involves the inhibition of the stimulus to point the hand to the number ten. Figure 2.1 shows a variety of clock test results ranging from intact to severely impaired.

Methods of clock test scoring are many and varied, but research suggests that the simpler the scoring system the better. A four-point scoring system records zero for an intact clock, one point for mild impairment, two points for moderate impairment and three points for severe impairment. This scoring system was recommended by the Consortium to Establish a Registry for Alzheimer's Disease (CERAD) (Figure 2.2). Borson and colleagues have incorporated the CDT in the Mini-Cog. The Mini-Cog uses a two-step process, including a test of delayed recall and the CDT (Figure 2.3).

A variant of the CDT known as the CLOX test is designed to detect frontal lobe/ executive impairment. In the first step (CLOX 1), the patient is asked to draw a free-hand clock. If the patient is unable to do this or cannot do it accurately, the patient is then asked to copy a drawing of a completed clock (CLOX 2). If the first component (CLOX 1) is impaired but CLOX 2 is intact (copying ability is retained), this suggests frontal lobe/executive impairment (Figure 2.4).

Qualitative assessment of clock drawing may be as useful as quantitative scoring. One can observe perseveration, poor planning and conceptual deficits from the CDT. Like other screening instruments, the CDT lends itself to use as a monitor of change over time especially because it is a simple visual record that can be readily compared from one visit to another.

Tests of Executive Function

The frontal lobes oversee a number of important functions, including concentration and attention, complex planning, response inhibition, switching between tasks, abstract thinking, insight, judgement and verbal fluency. The CDT in part depends upon intact executive function, although it casts a wide 'cognitive net' and also draws on other cognitive domains such as visuospatial function. However, other more specific tests may be easily incorporated into a cognitive screen. The frontal assessment battery (FAB) is designed specifically to detect frontal dysfunction. It includes six items measuring a range of frontal functions,

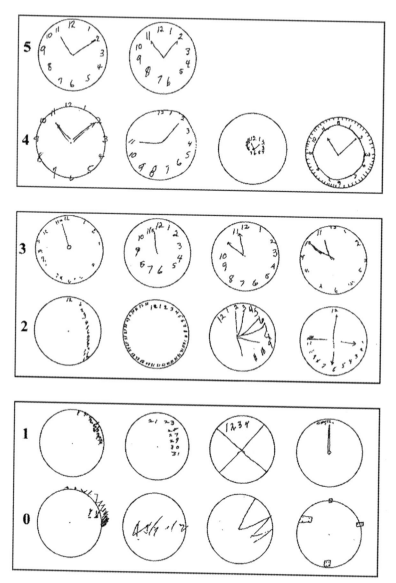

Figure 2.1 A variety of clock test results ranging from intact to severely impaired

including mental flexibility, abstract reasoning, inhibitory control, motor programming and environmental autonomy. These tests include (1) similarities; (2) verbal fluency; (3) Luria's three-step procedure (fist, edge, palm), a test of motor programming; (4) the use of conflicting instructions 'tap twice when I tap once' alternating with 'tap once when I tap twice'; (5) Go-no-go test (inhibitory control) 'tap once when I tap once' alternating with 'do not tap when I tap twice' and (6) prehension behaviour (environmental autonomy). In this test, the patient sits with palms faced upwards resting on the knees. The patient is instructed not to take the examiner's hands when the examiner touches the palm of the patient. In

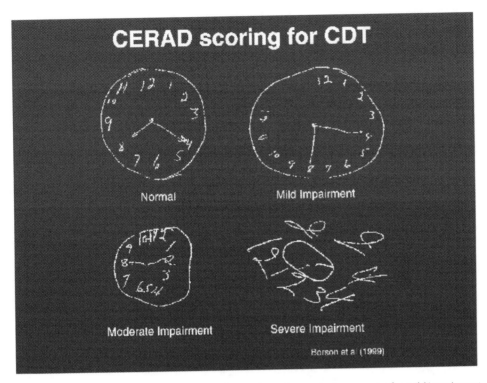

Figure 2.2 A four-point scoring system records zero for an intact clock, one point for mild impairment, two points for moderate impairment and three points for severe impairment
Reproduced from Borson *et al.* (1999), with permission from The Gerontological Society of America.

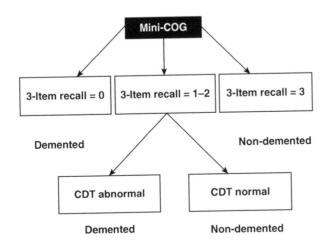

Figure 2.3 The Mini-Cog uses a two-step process, including a test of delayed recall and the clock-drawing test Reproduced from Borson *et al.* (2000), with permission from John Wiley & Sons Ltd.

CLOX Test

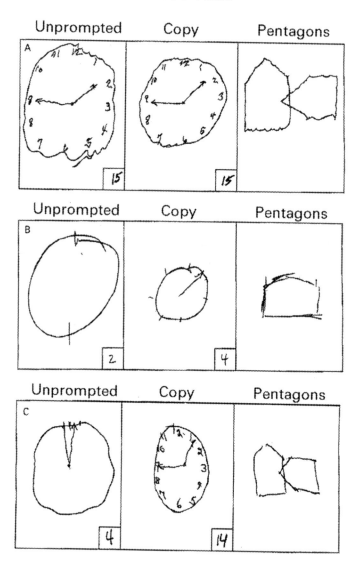

Figure 2.4 The CLOX test is designed to detect frontal lobe/executive impairment. In the first step (CLOX 1), the patient is asked to draw a free-hand clock. If the patient is unable to do this or cannot do it accurately, the patient is then asked to copy a drawing of a completed clock (CLOX 2). If the first component (CLOX 1) is impaired but CLOX 2 is intact (copying ability is retained), this suggests frontal lobe/executive impairment

Reproduced from Royall *et al.* (1998), with permission from the BMJ Publishing Group.

frontal lobe dysfunction the patient may be unable to resist grasping the examiner's hands even when instructed to the contrary.

Tasks that require shifts of mental set may reveal perseveration, a non-specific but sensitive sign of brain dysfunction. This can be tested by drawing three loops and asking the patient to copy these loops across the page. Patients with perseveration may add extra loops to the three that are recorded. One can also use a line of alternating triangles and rectangles to see if the patient can alternate between different patterns. In the 'go–no–go' sequence, the examiner taps twice and asks the patient to tap once and then asks the patient to tap twice when the examiner taps once. Using random tapping of one or two taps allows the determination whether the patient can adjust and switch sets accordingly, or if the patient lapses into a perseverative response by mimicking the number of taps the examiner makes. Abstract reasoning may be tested by asking about similarities such as 'how are a man and a tree alike', differences (e.g. 'what is the difference between a child and a dwarf') or the examiner may ask about the meaning of common proverbs (though responses to questions about proverbs are heavily dependent upon education and culture). Trail-making tasks, such as Trail A or Trail B, may be used to detect executive impairment and are brief-timed tests which may readily incorporated into any assessment. Verbal fluency in part depends upon intact executive function, and in a task of phonemic fluency one may ask the patient to list as many words as possible that begin with the letter F in 60 seconds. Performance on this task depends on expressive language abilities, but the individual may also benefit from a cognitive strategy, such as working through different vowels or letters of the alphabet sequentially, to generate more words. An alternate task of verbal fluency would be to 'name as many animals as you can in the 60 seconds'. This is called semantic or category fluency. It is often considered that patients with Alzheimer's disease who have mainly temporal lobe involvement may experience a greater decline in semantic or category fluency, while patients with primarily frontal lobe pathology may have particular difficulty with phonemic fluency.

Montreal Cognitive Assessment

The MoCA is one of the most commonly used brief cognitive tests. It was devised in part to address the deficiencies of previous cognitive tests that did not adequately assess executive function and represents an important advancement in this regard. It is more sensitive in mild cognitive impairment and a number of different language versions are available at www.mocatest.org. The MoCA contains some elements in common with the MMSE but also includes a test of phonemic fluency, clock drawing and a brief trail-making task, among others. It is scored out of 30, and a cut point of 26 was initially suggested as suitable to detect dementia. It has good sensitivity, but may have poor specificity using this cut point in mixed populations and so it has been suggested that a lower cut point may be more appropriate depending on the population under study. Performance on the MoCA is particularly dependent upon age and education. Normative population data have been published indicating a broad range of normative values according to age and educational level, but the requirement for users to undergo online training may affect its popularity.

Longer Cognitive Tests

In addition to the brief tests listed earlier in the chapter, there are a number of longer cognitive batteries that combine tests of several cognitive domains. The ACE, CAMCOG (Cambridge Cognitive Examination) and ADAS-Cog (Alzheimer's Disease Assessment Scale, cognitive subscale) are commonly used, the latter being utilised as a change measure in many drug trials. These tests take longer to administer but provide a more detailed assessment of specific cognitive domains and can be more sensitive to change over time. In circumstances where detailed neuropsychological evaluation is required (e.g. for mild disorders, when the presentation does not fit a typical pattern of impairment or when high intelligence and extensive education cause a patient to do well on short cognitive screens despite likely decline from a previous high level of function), the specialised input of a neuropsychologist is extremely helpful in eliciting the relative strengths and weaknesses of specific cognitive domains and in clarifying patterns of cognitive impairment to aid diagnosis. A typical neuropsychological evaluation will cover a wide range of cognitive functions and take around two hours (sometimes split over a couple of sessions to avoid the impact of fatigue) to complete. When language disorder is the predominant presenting symptom (e.g. in suspected Primary Progressive Aphasia), assessment by a speech pathologist can be most helpful.

Cognitive Testing and Capacity

Clinicians are often asked to make a determination regarding the decision-making capacity of an older adult. The general cognitive assessment, as described earlier, is relevant in capacity assessments as it provides a reflection of global cognitive functioning. However, it is important to note that decision-making capacity is considered 'task-specific' and includes two fundamental components: (1) an understanding of relevant facts, and (2) an appreciation of the consequences of taking or not taking a specific action. In this regard, an assessment of cognitive function although helpful, does not determine whether an individual does or does not have capacity. The range of capacity assessments that may be requested include the capacity to create a power of attorney, consent to treatment, decide where to reside or to make a will. In addition to the general cognitive screen, the clinician must ask questions that are specific and relevant to each of the capacities being assessed. This nearly always includes relevant information from key informants or caregivers. Of course, legal definitions of capacity may vary between jurisdictions.

Physical Examination

In addition to cognitive assessment, a focused physical examination is a routine component of an initial assessment in older adults. Typically, the examination is focused upon neurological features associated with underlying cognitive disorders. For example, motor or sensory deficits in the context of cerebrovascular disease or Parkinsonism in Lewy body disease. However, a broad range of general medical conditions may impact upon psychiatric disorders in later life. Many older adults have multiple comorbidities. It is important to detect these and to have a good understanding of how common conditions, such as cardiovascular disease, musculoskeletal and respiratory conditions, diabetes or other endocrine disorders, can interact with psychiatric disorders in older adults. For example, chronic pain or functional impairment may precipitate or exacerbate depression in an older adult (in community surveys urinary incontinence is strongly associated with depressive symptoms) and should therefore be addressed as part of a multidisciplinary care plan. In addition, safe prescribing is dependent upon good knowledge of how psychotropic medications interact with existing medical conditions and other prescribed medications. In most instances, effective management and treatment of psychiatric disorders in older adults involves working collaboratively with other healthcare professionals to address unmet healthcare needs in an integrated care plan as discussed further in subsequent sections.

Further Investigations

Most older adults with psychiatric symptoms or cognitive decline will undergo a basic battery of tests in order to rule out common, treatable conditions which may either be contributing to or causing the symptoms described. Tests to consider include a full blood examination (to look for anaemia, which might contribute to fatigue, macrocytosis, possibly indicative of alcohol excess or B12 deficiency, and neutrophilia or leukocytosis associated with infection or an underlying myeloproliferative disorder). Inflammatory markers, such as erythrocyte sedimentation rate, may be elevated in the context of vasculitis or other immune conditions, but are often non-specific. A renal profile is useful to exclude chronic kidney disease and determine if doses of medications primarily excreted by renal clearance require adjustment. Baseline sodium can help inform choice of antidepressant as serotonergic medications can precipitate or worsen hyponatraemia. Evaluation of liver enzymes is relevant for medications primarily metabolised in the liver and to detect significant alcohol abuse. Hypercalcaemia or hypothyroidism can be associated with depressed mood among other symptoms and 1 in 20 memory clinic attenders will have an abnormal thyroid-stimulating hormone result. Many physicians will screen for cardiovascular risk factors by checking glucose and lipid profile as these may result in increased cardiovascular morbidity and accelerated cognitive decline. B12 is routinely checked in older adults as deficiency can result in peripheral neuropathy and also cognitive decline. Although reversing mild B12 deficiency rarely results in significant cognitive improvement, an abnormal B12 result is found in around 5 per cent of attenders at memory clinics. Syphilis serology should be conducted only when there are known risk factors; a weakly positive result may raise more problems than it solves. In circumstances where there is an acute or chronic cognitive decline suggestive of delirium, routine investigations to exclude infection are requested. These will typically include a urine test, perhaps a chest X-ray (also worth doing when the patient is or has been a smoker) and routine haematological investigations. An ECG is useful to exclude underlying conduction abnormalities (e.g. prolonged QTc), which may be of relevance when prescribing certain psychotropic medications, including cholinesterase inhibitors and some antipsychotic and antidepressant medications, particularly in those with complicating cardiovascular disease or who use other medications which impact upon cardiac conduction.

In the context of cognitive decline, neuroimaging is routinely conducted to determine aetiology and exclude potentially reversible causes of cognitive decline. The type of neuro-imaging requested will depend on the circumstances and clinical question to be answered. For example, a CT brain scan may adequately exclude acute changes, such as a subdural in an older adult who has recently fallen, while an MRI will more sensitively detect micro-angiopathic disease in an individual with mild cognitive impairment and can detect hippocampal atrophy, which, if present, raises the likelihood of the presence of Alzheimer's disease and is associated with a faster rate of decline than if absent. In specialist centres when there is a change in behaviour or cognitive function that is otherwise unexplained by structural neuroimaging, functional modalities, such as PET or SPECT, may more sensitively detect regional changes in perfusion or metabolic activity in advance of structural changes. Molecular neuroimaging to determine whether an individual has a significant cerebral burden of amyloid or tau pathology is mostly confined to research settings at present, but if treatments, such as antibodies, can be developed which retard or delay progression of cognitive decline in people with preclinical or prodromal AD, amyloid imaging with PET may become widespread. Blood tests that correlate with cerebral amyloid and tau levels have been developed and may attain a clinical role in future. Similarly, measurement of CSF amyloid and tau levels is mostly of research interest to date, although in circumstances where there is an acute decline in cognition or evidence of delirium, CSF analysis may exclude infectious and autoimmune processes. Electroencephalography may be helpful if an underlying seizure disorder is considered likely or to detect periodic complexes frequently seen in Creutzfeldt Jacob disease. Genetic testing for dominantly inherited neurodegenerative disorders may be offered to individuals with or at risk of certain neurocognitive disorders and a suggestive family history after they and key family members have received appropriate genetic counselling.

Referral for Further Assessments

The availability of neuropsychologists, speech pathologists and occupational therapists varies markedly between and even within countries. Where available, neuropsychologists may assist greatly in the assessment of those with equivocal or unusual cognitive impairment, and those whose assessment is rendered more difficult by virtue of either very high education, unclear level of literacy, sensory impairment, language or cultural factors. Speech pathologists may assist with language assessment or remediation of language difficulties. An occupational therapist's assessment of function or driving often reveals more about domestic competence, home safety or risk to other road users than many hours of assessment in the office or clinic.

Conclusion

A thorough and well-documented initial assessment is the cornerstone of competent and effective care in POA. What goes unseen initially may remain undetected. The varied clinical presentations and high frequency of comorbid medical conditions in later life mandate a comprehensive initial assessment.

Further Reading

Articles

Borson, S. *et al.* (2000). The Mini-Cog: a cognitive 'vital signs' measure for dementia screening in multi-lingual elderly. *International Journal of Geriatric Psychiatry*, 15, 1021–1027. doi: 10.1002/1099-1166.

A useful screening test.

Brodaty, H. *et al.* (2002). The GPCOG: a new screening test for dementia designed for general practice. *Journal of the American Geriatrics Society*, 50, 530–534. doi: 10.1046/j.1532-5415.2002.50122.x.

A screening test designed for use in primary care.

Burns, A., Harrison, J. R., Symonds, C. and Morris, J. (2020). A novel hybrid scale for the assessment of cognitive and executive function: the Free-Cog. *International Journal of Geriatric Psychiatry*, 36, 566–572. doi: 10/1002/gps.5454.

An intriguing new scale that integrates measurement of cognition and executive function.

Folstein, M. F., Folstein, S. E. and McHugh, P. R. (1975). Mini-Mental State: a practical method for grading the cognitive state of patients for clinicians. *Journal of Psychiatric Research*, 12, 189–198. doi: 10.1016/0022-3956(75)90026-6.

The best known brief cognitive test.

Gallagher, D. *et al.* (2010). Late life depression: a comparison of risk factors and symptoms according to age of onset in community dwelling older adults. *International Journal of Geriatric Psychiatry*, 25, 981–987. doi: 10.1002/gps.2438.

Describes differences between depression with first onset in later life compared to early onset depression.

Kenny, R. A. *et al.* (2013). Normative values of cognitive and physical function in older adults: findings from the Irish Longitudinal Study on Ageing. *Journal of the American Geriatrics Society*, 61: Suppl 2, S279–S290. doi: 10.1111/jgs.12195.

Contains useful tables of normal population values for MMSE and MoCA according to age and educational level.

Kipps, C. M. and Hodges, J. R. (2005). Cognitive assessment for clinicians. *Journal of Neurology, Neurosurgery and Psychiatry*, 76: Suppl 1, i22–i30. doi: 10.1136/jnnp.2004.059758.

An excellent summary paper on this topic.

Nasreddine, Z. S. *et al.* (2005). The Montreal Cognitive Assessment, MoCA: a brief screening tool for mild cognitive impairment. *Journal of the American Geriatrics Society*, 53, 695–699. doi: 10.1111/j.1532-5415.2005.53221.x.

The MoCA is one of the most widely used cognitive tests.

Shulman, K. I. (2000). Clock-drawing: is it the ideal cognitive screening test? *International Journal of Geriatric Psychiatry*, 15, 548–561. doi: 10.1002/1099-1166(200006).

A thorough overview.

Shulman, K. I. *et al.* (2006). IPA survey of brief cognitive screening instruments. *International Psychogeriatrics*, 18, 281–294. doi: 10.1017/S1041610205002693.

As discussed previously, this survey found the MMSE to be the most popular test.

Storey, J. E. *et al.* (2004). The Rowland Universal Dementia Assessment Scale (RUDAS): a multicultural cognitive assessment scale. *International Psychogeriatrics*, 16, 13–31. doi: 10.1017/S1041610205003133.

Instrument designed for use in different linguistic and cultural groups, including individuals with limited formal education.

Velayudhan, L. *et al.* (2014). Review of brief cognitive tests for patients with suspected dementia. *International Psychogeriatrics*, 26, 1247–1262. doi: 10.1017/S1041610214000416.

Good descriptions of several brief cognitive tests.

Walterfang, M., Siu, R. and Velakoulis, D. (2006). The NUCOG: validity and reliability of a brief cognitive screening tool in neuropsychiatric patients. *Australian and New Zealand Journal of Psychiatry*, 40, 995–1002. doi: 10.1080/j.1440-1614.2006.01923.x.

A validated assessment instrument.

Books

Darzins, P., Molloy, D. W. and Strang, D. (2000). *Who Can Decide? The Six Step Capacity Assessment Process*. Adelaide: Memory Australia Press.

Excellent practical approach to an issue that is frequently encountered when working with older adults.

David, A., Fleminger, S., Kopelman, M., Lovestone, S. and Mellers, J. (2012). *Lishman's Organic Psychiatry*, 4th ed. Chichester: Wiley.

This classic text contains an excellent section on all aspects of clinical assessment.

Hodges, J. (2017). *Cognitive Assessment for Clinicians*, 3rd ed. Oxford: Oxford University Press.

Aims to teach how to assess cognition in the clinic and succeeds.

Chapter 3

Differential Diagnosis: The Three Ds

Introduction

This chapter addresses an approach to the differential diagnosis of the major syndromes encountered in the psychiatry of old age, namely the three Ds: depression, delirium and dementia. In terms of prevalence, these conditions represent the vast majority of psychiatric disorders encountered in the clinical psychiatry of late life, and hence, an approach to differential diagnosis is essential in terms of understanding and management. Particular attention is given in this chapter to the relationship between depression and dementia.

History Taking

As discussed in the previous chapter on assessment, history taking is one of the most important means by which we establish a diagnosis and differentiate various syndromes. Simply identifying the onset of the history of present illness can be most revealing. Most causes of dementia typically have an insidious, chronic and progressive course prior to the time of psychiatric assessment. Usually, this is in the order of years in duration. The onset of illness is distinctly different to delirium, in which onset is typically acute, developing over hours to days prior to medical attention. In between the two syndromes of dementia and delirium is major depression, whose onset tends to be sub-acute in nature, usually in the order of weeks to months. Hence, one could argue that a simple description of the timeline of the presenting symptoms can go a long way in differentiating the three Ds and establishing a provisional diagnosis. However, as highlighted in Chapter 6, the most common risk factor for the development of delirium is dementia or cognitive impairment of any kind. Thus, one may have both a delirium and dementia as well as comorbid depression with dementia. In older adults (as discussed in Chapter 2), it is routine to obtain information regarding cognitive symptoms and impact on function from a reliable informant, as a patient with cognitive impairment and limited insight will typically overestimate their abilities.

It often occurs that following an initial assessment, a number of differential diagnoses will be entertained. In that case, simply following the patient's clinical course and assessing the outcome will frequently reveal the true nature of the underlying condition. The dementias, or major neurocognitive disorders, by their very nature are degenerative conditions with a resultant progressive decline in cognition and function over time. Some patients with delirium will demonstrate a significant improvement in cognition and functioning following treatment of the underlying cause. However, not all patients with delirium will return to their pre-morbid functional level, and delirium is an important risk factor for the future development of an irreversible dementia.

As in younger populations, the clinical course of major depressive disorder is character-ised by a pattern of recovery and vulnerability to recurrence, often with periods of relatively good functioning between episodes. However, there is a significant overlap between cognitive impairment and depression in later life. Many older adults with depression, who do not have a diagnosis of dementia, will have cognitive deficits, particularly executive cognitive deficits, and meet criteria for mild cognitive impairment or mild neurocognitive disorder. Depression in early life variably has been associated with increased risk of dementia, and late life depression consistently has been associated with an approximately twofold increased risk of both vascular and Alzheimer's dementia. In the past, patients who presented with reversible cognitive deficits in the context of dementia were considered to have 'pseudo-dementia'. However, subsequent studies have demonstrated that the majority of patients initially considered to have 'pseudo-dementia' subsequently develop dementia if followed over a longer time. In most instances, cognitive deficits observed in the context of depression do not fully resolve following treatment and are associated with increased risk of functional decline over time. The 'vascular hypothesis' of depression proposes that frontos-triatal pathology, disconnecting frontal control structures from underlying striatal and limbic structures critical for regulation of mood, motivation and stress responses, can precipitate and perpetuate depression in older adults. There is evidence, therefore, to support a bidirectional relationship between depression and dementia, whereby depression itself may result in accelerated cognitive decline but may also occur as a consequence of cognitive impairment.

Medical History

A good understanding of medical comorbidity is critical when managing psychiatric disorders in older adults. In the context of dementia, medical status can vary widely, ranging from severely ill bedridden individuals to those who appear to be perfectly healthy, robust and independent in basic activities of daily living (bathing, dressing, walking) yet are dependent on others for support with instrumental activities of daily living (managing finances, medication or tasks requiring more complex decision mak-ing). It is particularly important to pay attention to modifiable risk factors for cognitive decline which should be addressed as part of a multidisciplinary care plan. Common modifiable risk factors include behavioural risk factors (e.g. excessive alcohol intake, smoking, physical inactivity), those related to specific medical conditions (e.g. hyper-tension that is poorly controlled or certain endocrine disorders) and medications which may exacerbate cognitive dysfunction (e.g. anticholinergic, opiate or benzodiazepine medication). Several medical conditions may precipitate depression (e.g. hypothyroid-ism or hypercalcaemia), and certain medical conditions may exacerbate or mimic aspects of the depressive syndrome (e.g. anaemia or sleep apnoea exacerbating fatigue). In circumstances where there is treatment resistance, it is particularly important to review the diagnosis and underlying medical conditions which may be contributing to persistence of symptoms.

In the context of delirium, there are ordinarily several contributory factors. A typical example might include a vulnerable older adult with mild cognitive impairment who falls, sustains a hip fracture and is therefore exposed to several potentially deliriogenic insults, including trauma, pain, infection and very possibly opiate analgesic medication. In such instances, a psychiatry service may be consulted to help clarify the diagnosis and advise

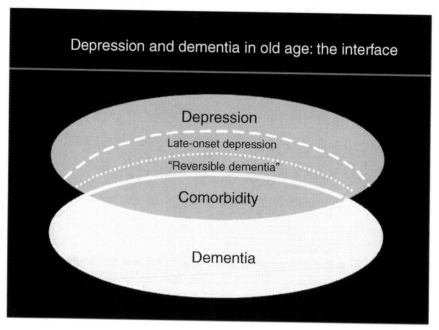

Figure 3.1 Depression and dementia in old age: the interface

regarding symptomatic management of agitation. Thorough investigation and treatment of underlying causes is central to the management of delirium. It is important to review and advise regarding all possible contributory factors in such instances (e.g. treating underlying infection, tapering or optimising the dose of potentially deliriogenic medications and addressing environmental risk factors, as discussed in Chapter 6).

Figures 3.1–3.3 illustrate the relationship between depression, dementia and reversible dementias, reflecting the prevalence of comorbidities and the shift over time from depressive syndromes to dementia.

Psychiatric and Family History

Commonly, psychiatrists working with older adults are asked to distinguish between a mood disorder and an evolving neurodegenerative condition. In such instances there may be one underlying diagnosis or two overlapping conditions. The clinical presentation and timeline of symptomatic expression will often help distinguish the two (see Table 3.1). Not uncommonly, apathy is misdiagnosed as depression in this population (see Table 3.2). It is important to remember that apathy can exist independent of depression and is often one of the earliest symptoms of an evolving neurodegenerative disorder. In these cases, the carer is often more concerned about the patient's amotivation, while the patient may appear indifferent with no other symptoms of depression. In such instances a personal or family history of depression may be less likely, while a positive family of dementia may be more likely. If depression occurs for the first time in late life, it is significantly more likely to be associated with cognitive decline and less likely to be associated with positive family history of depression when compared to

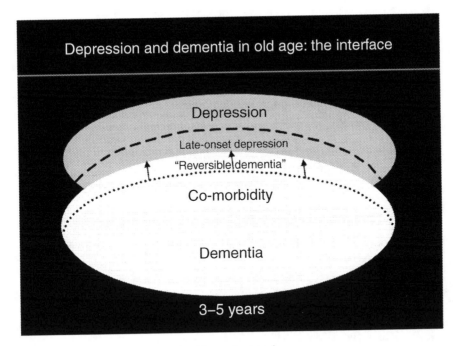

Figure 3.2 Depression and dementia in old age: the interface

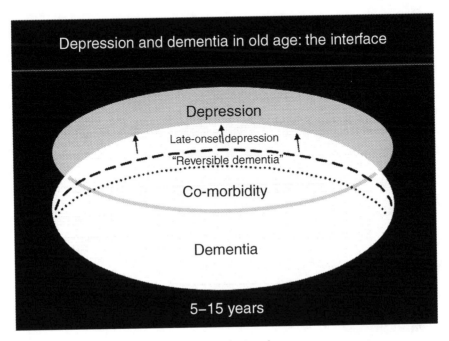

Figure 3.3 Depression and dementia in old age: the interface

Table 3.1 Differentiating the three Ds in the assessment of an older adult

	Dementia	Delirium	Depression
Onset	Insidious	Acute	Subacute
Course	Progressive Relapsing/Remitting	Acute fluctuations (hours/days)	(weeks/months)
Medical status	Variable	Acute illness/drug toxicity	Variable
Family history	Possible family history of dementia	Variable	Possible family history of mood disorder

Table 3.2 Common diagnostic pitfalls in the three Ds

Depression	Apathy may be misdiagnosed as depression
	Cognitive impairment in depression may be missed if cognition is not routinely assessed during initial consultation
Dementia	Cognitive assessment should assess memory but should also include an assessment of executive function commonly impaired in neuropsychiatric disorders
Delirium	Hyperactive or agitated delirium is more likely to be diagnosed while hypoactive delirium is commonly missed

those with early onset depression. It is important, therefore, that when behavioural symptoms emerge for the first time in late life, the treating physician retains a high index of suspicion for an underlying neurological disorder. Several population studies have now demonstrated that behavioural symptoms are often the first manifestation of an evolving neurocognitive disorder and that symptoms such as depression, anxiety and apathy are extremely common in mild cognitive impairment/mild neurocognitive disorder. Early recognition of an underlying neurocognitive disorder is important to help prevent further cognitive decline and has implications for treatments chosen to manage behavioural symptoms.

Examination

Mental state examination is a critical component for helping to differentiate between the three Ds in older adults. A patient with delirium typically will have a clouded sensorium with impaired attention, although this may fluctuate throughout the day. In contrast, patients with dementia or depression will have a clear sensorium and should be able to engage better with cognitive testing. Depression and cognitive impairment often impact upon attention, but this is typically less so than in a patient with acute delirium. An individual with depression may respond to questions with 'I don't know' or 'I don't care' answers while most patients with cognitive impairment, unless apathy is very prominent,

Table 3.3 Differential diagnosis of psychotic symptoms

	Dementia	Delirium	Depression
Delusions	Compensatory	Nightmarish	Nihilistic
Hallucinations	Variable	Visual	Auditory
Content	Persecutory/ Theft/infidelity	Frightening bizarre	Self-deprecatory

will make effortful but incorrect responses. In addition, patients with depression will have all of the affective characteristics of an individual with depression, with associated negative cognitions regarding the world, self and future. Delusional content in depression is typically nihilistic or self-deprecatory (see Table 3.3), while common delusional themes in cognitive disorders include delusions of theft, persecution or infidelity. Visual hallucinations are typically associated with delirium although they can occur in dementia, particular dementia with Lewy bodies, where visual hallucinations may be an early feature. Physical assessment in certain neurocognitive disorders such as early Alzheimer's disease may be unremarkable, while cerebrovascular disease or Parkinson's will impact on gait and balance earlier in the disease process. The physical assessment in depression will depend upon the underlying aetiological process with many patients with so-called vascular depression presenting with a dysexecutive syndrome on cognitive testing and some impairment of gait or balance on neurological examination.

Further Reading

Articles

Alexopoulos, G. S. et al. (1993). The course of geriatric depression with 'reversible dementia': a controlled study. *American Journal of Psychiatry*, 150, 1693–1699. doi: 10.1176/ajp.150.11.1693.

A classic follow-up study of patients with what was once termed 'depressive pseudo-dementia'.

Butters, M. A. et al. (2008). Pathways linking late-life depression to persistent cognitive impairment and dementia. *Dialogues in Clinical Neuroscience*, 10, 345–357. doi: 10.31887/DCNS.2008.10.3/mabutters.

An excellent overview of mechanisms linking depression with cognitive decline.

Gallagher, D. et al. (2017). Neuropsychiatric symptoms in mild cognitive impairment. An update on prevalence, mechanisms, and clinical significance. *Canadian Journal of Psychiatry*, 62, 161–169. doi: 10.1177/0706743716648296.

Review of neuropsychiatric symptoms before and after onset of mild cognitive impairment.

Taylor, W. D. et al. (2013). The vascular depression hypothesis: mechanisms linking vascular disease with depression. *Molecular Psychiatry*, 18, 963–974. doi: 10.1038/mp.2013.20.

Review of the vascular depression hypothesis incorporating more recent mechanistic theories.

Book chapters

Shulman, K. I. and Silver, I. L. (2006). Assessment of older adults. In D. Goldbloom, (ed.). *Psychiatric Clinical Skills*, Philadelphia, PA: Elsevier Mosby, pp 315–325.

Recommended reading for aspiring old age psychiatrists and geriatricians.

<table>
<tr><td>**Chapter**
4</td><td># The Dementias</td></tr>
</table>

Dementia Defined

Definitions of dementia have been getting longer and more complex, and recently the term itself has come under challenge. Seventy years ago, a leading psychiatric textbook defined dementia in one short sentence. Current diagnostic manuals devote pages to its definition. Tables 4.1 and 4.2 give summaries of the diagnostic criteria used by the World Health Organisation's ICD-11 and the American Psychiatric Association's DSM-5 systems, which are the criteria that will be most used in clinical practice and research during the lifetime of this edition. Because ICD-11 will retain the term 'dementia', and it is an international classification rather than a purely American one, and because the new DSM-5 appellation of Major Cognitive Disorder has not gained universal acceptance, we continue to use the term 'dementia' in this edition. Strict application of the different criteria will yield different rates of dementia in any population assessed because the criteria differ in the levels of impairment required to diagnose it. However, all definitions of dementia include certain core features. First, dementia is a *syndrome* (a collection of symptoms and signs) with multiple causes. Second, dementia is an *acquired* condition and represents a *decline* from a previous level of function no matter how exalted or limited that level of function used to be. Third, the diagnosis can be made only in an *alert* patient because one important differential diagnosis is delirium, which is characterised by both cognitive impairment and an impaired level of consciousness. Fourth, while memory impairment is usually present, dementia affects not only memory but *multiple* higher mental functions such as intellect and personality. Last, dementia is not a diagnosis based solely on the patient's performance in an unfamiliar testing setting but must be rooted in real-world problems: namely, impairment of *social or occupational functioning*. Reversible dementia syndromes exist, and some dementias can present with static impairments that do not get worse, but most cases of dementia are irreversible and progressive.

Types and Causes of Dementia

Table 4.3 lists a large number of causes of dementia, including conditions that may present with an apparent dementia syndrome. However, most such presentations are not encountered in clinical practice very often. Alzheimer's disease (AD), vascular dementia (VaD), mixed vascular and Alzheimer's disease, dementia with Lewy bodies (DLB), frontotemporal dementia (FTD) and dementia associated with alcohol-related brain damage are the most common types of dementia.

Table 4.1 ICD-11 diagnostic criteria for dementia (abbreviated)

Dementia is an acquired brain syndrome characterised by a decline from a previous level of cognitive functioning with impairment in two or more cognitive domains (such as memory, executive functions, attention, language, social cognition and judgement, psychomotor speed and visuoperceptual or visuospatial abilities). The cognitive impairment is not entirely attributable to normal ageing and significantly interferes with independence in the person's performance of activities of daily living. Based on available evidence, the cognitive impairment is attributed or assumed to be attributable to a neurological or medical condition that affects the brain, trauma, nutritional deficiency, chronic use of specific substances or medications or exposure to heavy metals or other toxins.

Exclusions
Coma, delirium, disorders of intellectual development, neurodevelopmental disorders, stupor, old age.

ICD-11 gives separate detailed definitions for each of the following:
- Dementia due to Alzheimer's disease
- Dementia due to cerebrovascular disease
- Dementia due to Lewy body disease
- Frontotemporal dementia
- Dementia due to psychoactive substances
- Dementia due to diseases classified elsewhere
- Behavioural or psychological disturbances in dementia
- Dementia due to other specified cause and
- Dementia due to unknown or unspecified cause.

Source: World Health Organisation. (2018). *International Classification of Diseases (11th Revision)*. Retrieved from https://icd.who.int/en, 21 February 2021.
Readers should refer to the original document for the full criteria.

Table 4.2 DSM-5 criteria for major neurocognitive disorder (abbreviated)

- There is evidence of substantial cognitive decline from a previous level of performance in one or more of domains (Learning and memory, Language, Executive function, Complex attention, Perceptual-motor, Social cognition) based on the concerns of the individual, a knowledgeable informant or the clinician, and a decline in neurocognitive performance, typically involving test performance in the range of two or more standard deviations below appropriate norms (i.e. below the third percentile) on formal testing or equivalent clinical evaluation.
- The cognitive deficits are sufficient to interfere with independence (i.e. requiring minimal assistance with instrumental activities of daily living).
- The cognitive deficits do not occur exclusively in the context of a delirium.
- The cognitive deficits are not primarily attributable to another mental disorder (e.g. major depressive disorder and schizophrenia).

Source: American Psychiatric Association (2013). *Diagnostic and Statistical Manual of Mental Disorders, 5th ed.* Arlington, VA: American Psychiatric Association.

Table 4.3 Causes of the dementia syndrome

Neurodegenerative
Alzheimer's disease
Dementia with Lewy bodies
Parkinson's disease
Frontal and frontotemporal dementias

Vascular
Infarction(s)
Haemorrhage
Cardiovascular disease
Binswanger's encephalopathy
Vasculitis

Endocrine disorders
Diabetes
Hypo- or hyperthyroidism
Parathyroid disease
Cushing's disease
Addison's disease

Vitamin deficiencies
B12, thiamine (B1) and nicotinic acid

Systemic diseases
Severe respiratory disease
Anaemia

Other disorders of metabolism
Hyper- or hypocalcaemia
Severe liver disease

Neurological disorders and trauma
'Normal pressure' hydrocephalus
Head injury
Space-occupying lesions (e.g. tumours, haematomas)
Multiple sclerosis

Infections
Syphilis
Viral encephalitis
HIV
Creutzfeldt–Jakob disease

Substance use, abuse or withdrawal
Drugs
Alcohol

Psychiatric syndromes
Severe depression
Mania
Schizophrenia

Alzheimer's Disease

First described in the early twentieth century, AD is a progressive neurodegenerative disorder characterised pathologically by the presence of amyloid plaques between cortical neurones and neurofibrillary tangles within them. The occipital and motor cortices are relatively spared, while the lesions and associated atrophy tend to develop first in the entorhinal cortex and hippocampus before spreading throughout the temporal, parietal and frontal lobes. The plaques are aggregations of insoluble amyloid $A\beta42$ protein, a breakdown product of amyloid precursor protein (APP), which is a ubiquitous protein that may have a role in cell surface membrane reception. The tangles are comprised of hyperphosphorylated tau protein and represent the damaged remains of neurotubules, which are essential for the transport of nutrients to the extensive dendrites and axons of these neurones. In AD, a slow cascade of events occurring over up to 30 years leads to damage to dendritic connections and death of neurones. Although the disease process is asymptomatic in its early years, ultimately this damage destroys enough cellular connections to produce the characteristic symptoms of impaired new learning, dyspraxia, dysphasia, loss of judgement and, eventually, the complete loss of higher mental functions and the utter dependency of the affected individual. Death results from pneumonia associated with debility if no other comorbid disease process claims the life of the affected patient before this stage is reached.

Although some uncertainties about the nature of the pathological processes driving AD remain, the amyloid protein produced from APP plays a key role in initiating inflammatory processes that damage neurones and set off the accumulation of tangles and progressive neuronal loss.

Depending on the exact diagnostic criteria used, AD accounts for, or is a major contributory cause in, between 50 per cent and 80 per cent of all dementias. Risk factors for AD include advancing age, a family history of AD and the possession of the $\epsilon4$ allele of the lipid transport protein Apolipoprotein E (ApoE). Rare mutations in the APP gene on chromosome 21, the presenilin 1 gene on chromosome 14 and the presenilin 2 gene on chromosome 1 cause dominantly inherited familial AD with onset between age 40 and 60. Although these familial dementias account for only 1 per cent of all AD, the fact that these genes all produce proteins with a key role in the production of $A\beta42$ amyloid is a key piece of evidence in support of the 'amyloid hypothesis' of AD causation.

Vascular Dementia

A variety of manifestations of cerebrovascular disease, ranging from a single large cortical infarction to multiple small infarcts, down to subtle white matter changes due to small vessel ischaemia and resultant hypoperfusion, can produce a dementia syndrome. The symptoms of dementia seen in people with cerebrovascular disease depend on the nature of the underlying damage, but often frontal features, such as lack of initiative, are prominent, as are mood symptoms, especially depressed mood. Deficits tend to be patchy and unequal, onset usually is abrupt and progression is more likely to be stepwise or intermittent rather than steady and inexorable. Diagnostic criteria for VaD emphasise the presence of focal neurological signs (which may be transient), the presence of infarction in structural images obtained with CT or MRI and/or the presence of significant white matter changes affecting at least 25 per cent of the white matter. However, evidence is growing for more subtle changes associated with cerebral small vessel disease which may help identify this process at an earlier stage.

Mixed Vascular and Alzheimer Dementia

In autopsy series, the presence of at least some degree of cerebrovascular disease is common in the brains of those diagnosed as having AD during life. In addition, at least some pathological changes typical of AD are found in the brains of over 90 per cent of VaD patients who undergo a post-mortem brain examination. The fact that vascular risk factors, such as hypertension, diabetes, hypercholesterolaemia, smoking, obesity and lack of exercise, are associated with both VaD and AD in some studies may be due to these factors having some direct effect on APP metabolism or could suggest that subtle cerebrovascular arteriosclerosis can ensure that the symptomatic phase of AD is manifest earlier in those with AD pathology that might not yet be sufficient to produce cognitive impairment on its own.

Dementia with Lewy Bodies (DLB)

Early in the twentieth century, Friedrich Lewy described inclusion bodies in the neurones of the brain stem of individuals affected by Parkinson's disease. In the early 1990s, the microscopic examination of the cortical regions of some patients with primary progressive dementias revealed the presence of ubiquitin staining Lewy bodies in these regions too. Retrospective analysis of case records and subsequent prospective research indicate that individuals with primary progressive dementias who manifest any two of markedly fluctuating cognitive impairments, spontaneous motor Parkinsonism, visual hallucinations in clear consciousness and/or rapid eye movement (REM) sleep disorder are highly likely to exhibit cortical Lewy bodies at autopsy. Current international diagnostic criteria mandate a diagnosis of probable DLB when two in four of these features are present and possible DLB when only one clinical feature is present. Supportive clinical features are: severe sensitivity to antipsychotic agents, postural instability, repeated falls, syncope or other transient episodes of unresponsiveness, severe autonomic dysfunction (constipation, orthostatic hypotension, or urinary incontinence), hypersomnia, hyposmia, hallucinations in other modalities, systematised delusions, apathy, anxiety and depression. Indicative (reduced dopamine transporter uptake in basal ganglia demonstrated by SPECT/PET, abnormal 123I-MIBG myocardial scintigraphy and polysomnographic confirmation of REM sleep without atonia) and supportive (relative preservation of medial temporal lobe structures on CT/MRI, low uptake on SPECT/PET perfusion/metabolism scan with reduced occipital activity with/without the cingulate island sign on FDG-PET imaging, and prominent posterior slow-wave activity on EEG) biomarkers have been proposed. Most DLB patients are exquisitely sensitive to the extrapyramidal side effects of antipsychotic drugs, but when hallucinations create distress, some patients tolerate and are helped by atypical antipsychotics such as quetiapine or olanzapine. DLB sits on a disease spectrum with Parkinson's disease. The initial symptomatic manifestation of underlying pathology may be either motor or cognitive depending on the distribution of the lesions that characterise these conditions. If the first symptoms are motor rather than cognitive, and dementia first occurs at least one year following onset of parkinsonism then a diagnosis of Parkinson's disease dementia (PDD) rather than DLB is applied. However, this distinction is somewhat arbitrary.

Frontotemporal Dementias

A wide spectrum of pathologies producing progressive dementias that affect primarily the frontal or temporal lobes has been described. Frontotemporal dementia (FTD) tends to impact at a younger age than AD, and there is a family history in between 20 and 50 per cent of cases. They are characterised by pathologic accumulation of tau, TDP-43 or fused in sarcoma (FUS) proteins depending on the underlying subtype. In up to 60 per cent of familial cases, an underlying genetic mutation may be detected. The most common of these are in the C9orf72 gene on chromosome 9, the progranulin (PGN) or microtubule-associated protein tau (MAPT) genes on chromosome 17.

The clinical presentation is determined by the initial focus of degeneration in the brain. There is a behavioural variant that involves primarily the frontal lobe and three well-described language variants or primary progressive aphasias. In the behavioural variant, involvement of the inferior frontal lobes can result in disinhibited behaviours that cause embarrassment to others and may put the person with dementia at risk of injury or assault. Social judgement and safety awareness are often poor with ensuing risk-taking behaviours (e.g. dangerous driving). There is frequent loss of empathy, and as frontal dementias progress, apathy, produced by damage to the motivation centres in the inter-hemispheric fissure, becomes the most prominent feature until almost complete inanition supervenes. The most recent diagnostic criteria for behavioural-variant FTD are the Racovsky criteria. There is an overlap between the behavioural variant of FTD and motor neurone disease (MND), with up to one in seven patients with the behavioural variant developing MND. Three language-based variants or primary progressive aphasias have been described. Posterior frontal lobe damage affecting parts of the brain involved in language production may result in an expressive dysphasia, or there may be relative preservation of language fluency but loss of verbal knowledge in a semantic variant that primarily impacts the temporal neocortex in the early stage. A third language variant called the 'logopenic subtype' also has been described and is of some interest because it has been more commonly associated with underlying Alzheimer's rather than tau-based neuropathology.

Dementias Associated with Alcohol Abuse

End-organ vulnerability to the adverse effects of chronic overconsumption of alcohol varies markedly in respect of the liver and heart, and the same is true of the brain. Thiamine deficiency is a key mechanism in damage to the brain associated with overuse of alcohol, though the extent to which alcohol produces direct neurotoxicity is controversial. Typically, temporal (memory) and frontal functions are affected to the greatest degree in dementias associated with alcohol. There is prominent and often irreversible loss of short-term memory in the well-described Wernicke–Korsakoff syndrome. Other individuals may present with primarily executive cognitive difficulties, which can stabilise or improve with cessation of alcohol.

Other Uncommon Dementias

For detailed descriptions of uncommon dementias, the reader is referred to the list of further reading at the chapter's end. Dementia associated with syphilis, once very common, is now rare and tends to be characterised by disinhibition. Dementia associated with AIDS is a late manifestation of infection with HIV; more effective anti-retroviral treatments for HIV are associated with reduced risk of HIV-associated dementia, but once dementia is established, most such patients have a limited life expectancy.

Mild Cognitive Impairment

Mild cognitive impairment (MCI) is a term first coined by North American researchers to identify people at high risk of developing AD. This syndrome has been included in both DSM-5 and ICD-11 as mild neurocognitive disorder (MNCD). Use of the terms MCI and MNCD is now commonplace as clinicians see more and more such patients as the population ages and awareness of the treatability of some forms of dementia grows. It is characterised by cognitive decline, but critically the patient must retain functional independence and the condition is distinguished from a dementia syndrome or major neurocognitive disorder in this way. Expectations of 'independence' vary, which has led to uncertainty and ambiguity around the MCI concept. MCI is often defined arbitrarily as performance 1.5 standard deviations below the age- and education-adjusted norm on at least one neuropsychological test, where activities of daily living are substantially unimpaired, and there is concern regarding cognitive decline by either the person with the memory problem, a clinician or a close relative. Amnestic (affecting memory alone), non-amnestic and multi-domain forms of MCI are described. In reality, they constitute a heterogeneous group of disorders, but the underlying cause of MCI or MNCD may be determined by paying careful attention to clinical features together with use of neuroimaging or other biomarkers. For example, when MCI is present together with a positive Alzheimer's biomarker (positive amyloid PET scan or CSF sample with high tau and low $A\beta42$ levels), a diagnosis of prodromal AD or MCI due to AD may be given. Subjects diagnosed with MCI should be followed regularly, as up to 15 per cent (depending on the criteria used and the population from which the individuals are drawn) will develop dementia due to AD with each passing year, although a proportion may never decline and some even improve. Strategies that may attenuate decline in people with MCI include good control of vascular risk factors such as hypertension and 150 minutes per week of moderate-intensity physical exercise (such as brisk walking), social engagement and intellectual activity. Despite several disappointing trial results, work continues on anti-amyloid, anti-tau and other novel therapeutic approaches that it is hoped may prevent decline to dementia in the future.

The Epidemiology of Dementia

Dementia is common and becoming more so. The reason for this is simple. Dementia is an age-related disorder – the chances of being affected by dementia doubles every five years between the ages of 60 and 90 – and the world's population is ageing rapidly. There were around 50 million people with dementia in the world in 2020 and over 132 million are expected by 2050. Most of these people live in developing countries. All societies, races and cultures that have been studied have been found to contain people with dementia, but comparative epidemiology has not determined with certainty whether people living in one country or people from particular parts of the world are especially at risk of or uniquely protected against dementia.

The main unmodifiable risk factors for dementia are age, family history of dementia, female sex and the possession of one or more *ApoE* ε4 alleles (one of which trebles the risk of dementia developing at any age). Modifiable risk factors include years of education, hearing loss, excess alcohol use, hypertension, a head injury with post-traumatic amnesia exceeding one hour, obesity, smoking, air pollution, depression, physical inactivity, social isolation and diabetes. Vascular risk factors appear to increase the risk of both vascular dementia and AD. While most dementias manifest in late life, a small but important minority of people develop dementia in mid-adulthood and their needs and problems are rather different from those of old people with dementia. More than half of such early onset cases carry rare genetic mutations (usually dominantly inherited), causative of early onset dementia, including mutations in genes that affect APP processing (leading to early onset AD) and the tau gene (which can lead to early onset FTD). Although dominantly inherited dementias account for only about 1 per cent of all dementias, specialist genetic counselling and testing services are required to assist such families. Services for people with younger onset dementia need to cater for a very vulnerable group of patients, whose relatives are stressed by the decline of a family member in what should be the prime of life. Such services should be distinct, and are best organised at a regional level, because of the relatively small number of such patients in any one area.

The Symptoms and Natural History of Dementia

Mild

Although the initial and subsequent symptoms of dementia will depend upon the nature of the underlying disease process causing it, the majority of cases are due to AD, so the symptoms of this illness form the basis for the descriptions in this section.

Most people diagnosed with dementia present because their relatives are concerned, rather than because they themselves have insight into their deficits, though this may change with increased awareness of both dementia and the fact that some forms are treatable to a degree. Forgetfulness of recent events, missing appointments, diminishing ability to manage one's affairs and some degree of social withdrawal and declining motivation are common early features. Sometimes a person with dementia presents soon after their spouse, who had been assisting the person to a greater extent than others had realised, has died or had to leave home due to illness.

Assessment of those with mild dementia usually reveals rapid forgetting of newly learned information and may also detect mild nominal dysphasia, dyscalculia, constructional dyspraxia, rigidity of thought and some impairment of judgement. Progression tends to be slow, and if the affected individual receives a cognitive enhancer, there may be some months of improved performance before deterioration resumes and the individual reverts to and then passes their initial baseline. The phase of mild dementia may last for months or years, but in the typical 10-year course of an average case of AD, 2–5 years is likely to be spent in this phase of illness.

Many people with mild dementia can be left alone safely for hours, and some manage alone at home with support. Getting lost in familiar places is unusual when dementia is mild and sometimes driving ability is retained in the early stages, depending on the subtype and cognitive domains impacted, although all patients with dementia will have to stop driving eventually as the disease progresses. Although less attention may be paid to keeping one's person and home neat and tidy than was formerly the case, people with mild dementia can bathe, dress and use the lavatory without assistance. However, more complex activities, such as handling finances or engaging in paid employment, tend to be impaired.

Moderate

Whereas a person with mild dementia may appear unimpaired to a casual observer, the fact that impairments are present is readily apparent soon after meeting someone with moderate dementia. Household tasks, medication use and finances will need to be managed by another person. Some difficulties with dressing may be apparent, especially in regard to the use of catches, hooks, zips and buttons, and clothes will not be changed without prompting. Bathing will need to be encouraged and may require direct supervision. Inappropriate, disturbed and disturbing behaviours are common (see Chapter 5), and the patient cannot be left unsupervised for more than a few minutes. Some family members may no longer be recognised, though some personal information and the sense of self are likely to be retained. This phase may last from one to five years.

Severe

The patient with severe dementia is dependent upon others for even basic activities such as dressing, bathing, toileting and often eating as well. Continence is lost, language is restricted or lost entirely and constant supervision is required. In the final stages of dementia mobility goes and unless preventive action is taken, contractures and bedsores develop. Many people with dementia die of vascular disease and cancers, but deaths due to both accidents and pneumonia are more common in those with dementia than among the rest of the population. Although people with severe dementia who are cared for well sometimes live for up to a decade, death from pneumonia usually occurs within one to three years.

Assessment and Diagnosis

All too often dementia presents late in the course of the disorder when valuable opportunities to prevent crises and forestall entry to residential care have been lost. Early referral to specialist services should be encouraged and such services must be equipped to diagnose and manage mild dementia as well as more advanced cases.

Although this section describes some of the specific features of an assessment aimed at determining the presence of absence of a dementia syndrome, the reader should refer to Chapters 2 and 3 for additional information on this topic.

Informant History

Although some people in the early stages of dementia present to doctors with concerns about their memory, in most cases it is family members who initiate the process of assessment and diagnosis. The most important element of the initial assessment is obtaining a history from an informant who knows the patient well. If the patient and informant are to be seen by the same practitioner, then it shows greater respect to the patient if the informant interview takes place second. However, in many specialist clinics an informant interview is undertaken by a nurse or allied health professional, while a medical practitioner sees the patient. Although the patient's permission should be sought, the best way to conclude the initial consultation is to give some feedback about the findings of the assessment both to the patient and to the person(s) who accompany them to the consultation together.

In the informant interview, it is important to allow time for the story to emerge and the interviewee to explain the situation and to raise areas of concern, but some formal questioning will be necessary. The nature and extent of any cognitive deficits together with information about their impact on the patient's life should be determined. Any difficulties in everyday life, such as getting lost, problems managing medications, finances and shopping, should be enquired about. If the patient drives, the informant's opinion of their driving competence should be sought: 'Would you let your children drive with him/her?' is a useful question. Financial competence and whether the patient has a current will and/or an enduring power of attorney (EPOA) in place should be determined. As well as information about past medical history and current medications, any family history of dementia needs to be elicited. Behavioural and psychological symptoms of dementia form a separate chapter of this book, but they must be routinely enquired about at the initial informant interview. Finally, because stress, distress, depression and anxiety are common in the carers of those who have dementia, gentle enquiry as to the effect of the patient's symptoms upon the informant and how the informant is feeling about and managing the situation is an essential component of this assessment.

Medical Assessment

A history about the presenting complaint should be elicited from the patient, though often a lack of insight about some or all of the many problems in living that the patient is encountering will mean that they do not see why they need to be assessed. In these circumstances tact, compassion and diplomacy are required! Detailed personal and family histories should be obtained in addition to past and current medical history.

Screening for depressive and anxiety symptoms may be done with a standard questionnaire or by direct probing. At a bare minimum, cognitive assessment should utilise at least one standard screening instrument such as the Mini-mental State Examination, Montreal Cognitive Assessment, GPCOG, Mini-Cog or Abbreviated Mental Test Score. Depending on what is found, such tests may need to be supplemented with additional tests of memory (e.g. sentence recall, general knowledge), language function, praxis and frontal function. Sometimes, especially when no neuropsychologist is available, a longer cognitive assessment instrument, such as the Addenbrooke's Cognitive Examination, ADAS-Cog or CAMCOG, may be utilised. References for useful cognitive assessment instruments are provided at the end of Chapter 2.

It is essential to review all prescribed medications with a particular emphasis on those that may depress CNS function or that have anticholinergic properties.

Physical examination should be thorough and must include cardiovascular, respiratory, gastrointestinal and neurological components. Many people with dementia have comorbid medical conditions and sometimes these have not been diagnosed before and/or are not receiving appropriate treatment.

Neuropsychological Testing

Assessment by a neuropsychologist can be invaluable when cognitive impairment is mild or does not conform to an expected pattern, especially when the patient is younger than most. A neuropsychological assessment can take from one to three hours and will utilise standard tests appropriate for assessment of any deficits the patient may manifest. Not all patients with dementia need to be seen by a neuropsychologist, but it is impossible to offer a comprehensive dementia and cognitive assessment service if no neuropsychologist is available.

Special Investigations

It is more common to detect treatable comorbid disease than to find a reversible cause for dementia when special tests are ordered. Many of the investigations listed here will have been performed by a GP before the patient arrives for specialist assessment, and it is important that duplication of tests be avoided for reasons of cost and patient discomfort.

Most specialists request full blood examination (to rule out anaemia and rarer blood disorders), B12 and folate levels (most deficiencies found are mild and will not be the main cause of the cognitive impairment, but should be treated to prevent future problems), erythrocyte sedimentation rate (some dementias are caused by vasculopathies), liver function tests (these may reveal hitherto unsuspected alcohol abuse), electrolytes, creatinine and urea (to rule out renal impairment), thyroid-stimulating hormone (thyroid disease is common in late life) and glucose (and HbA1C in known diabetics), and we advocate measuring calcium and phosphate as well.

An ECG should be performed, especially if prescription of a cholinesterase inhibitor is contemplated, as uncorrected heart block is a contraindication to the prescription of a cholinergic drug.

Structural neuroimaging, such as a CT or an MRI, is often helpful to determine the extent of any cerebrovascular pathology or to rule out other considerations in patients with relevant risk factors. For example, it may be necessary to rule out metastatic disease in patients with a history of cancer, subdural or subarachnoid haemorrhage in patients with a history of traumatic brain injury or normal pressure hydrocephalus in those with associated neurological symptoms such as gait disturbance or urinary incontinence. The nature and extent of regional atrophy can help determine the underlying neurodegenerative aetiology. Pronounced hippocampal atrophy is strongly supportive of an AD diagnosis. Sometimes a scan can be used as an educational tool to assist the patient's family in understanding the organic nature of the changes they have observed in their affected relative (e.g. relating cerebral atrophy to decline in performance).

The use of more specialised tests, such as syphilis serology, autoantibody tests or EEGs, may be reserved for those with underlying risk factors or specific clinical features. Functional imaging modalities, such as SPECT, FDG PET and fMRI, may be helpful in specialised settings where structural scans have been inconclusive or demonstrate minimal changes in early disease, and can be useful in determining the brain region affected by the dementia, but most patients do not require such images. Molecular imaging techniques, such as amyloid PET, may move from being mostly a research-based tool to a routine investigation if anti-amyloid therapies are shown to be effective in preventing functional decline. There is also the potential for blood tests for AD, with researchers investigating the utility of p-tau 181 and p-tau 217. The potential benefits of novel testing modalities must be weighed against concerns regarding clinical applicability, cost and insurance and privacy concerns.

Managing the Person with Dementia and Their Carers

Imparting the Diagnosis

Telling someone that they have dementia is a heavy responsibility and it should be done with compassion, honesty and sufficient time available to answer questions and to discuss the implications. As most people with dementia have family or friends who will end up providing some care to them, and because it is common for family members to urge them to attend an assessment, the preferred method of imparting the diagnosis is in the setting up of a family meeting in which both the patient and significant others (e.g. spouse, children) are present. The recent COVID-19 pandemic has had a major deleterious impact upon the ability of clinicians to work in this way.

Although honesty is important, hope should not be extinguished. Some treatments are helpful in some dementias, and all people with dementia have the potential to benefit from social support and education of their families.

Some of the issues that need to be addressed include precise diagnosis, its prognosis and the potential benefits and risks of any treatment. Driving should be discussed at an early stage (most people with dementia who wish to continue to drive will need a formal driving assessment) and issues such as wills and EPOAs should be discussed. Most countries have Alzheimer's associations or societies that provide advice, support and education to people with dementia and their carers, and provision of contact details and encouragement to get in touch with the local association should be a key outcome of this meeting.

The imparting of a dementia diagnosis may cause distress that may make it hard for the recipient of the diagnosis and their family to remember all that has been discussed. For this reason, the provision of written feedback is essential, and in routine practice it is common for questions and discussion about the diagnosis, prognosis and management strategies to form the topic of an ongoing dialogue between patient, family and the treating team for many months or years. The provision of formal post-diagnostic support is important and should cover: (1) understanding the illness and managing its symptoms; (2) supporting community connections; (3) peer support; (4) planning for future decision making; and (5) planning for future care.

Although many general practitioners (GPs) take a strong interest in dementia and are highly competent in its management, it is often the case that the initial diagnosis will be made in a specialist setting, with some or all of the ongoing responsibility for management reverting to the GP after that has been done. It is helpful to both patient and family if specialists remain available for future consultation and advice after the initial diagnosis has been made and the management plan decided upon. Such availability also assists with the education of GPs, who may have received limited formal training about dementia.

Comorbid Medical Conditions

It is important that comorbid medical conditions, whether diagnosed previously or at the time of the dementia assessment, be optimally managed by the patient's GP and any medical specialists involved with care. In particular, vascular risk factors should be managed assertively to limit any potential vascular contribution to the dementia. Previously prescribed and any new medications will need to be supervised by a responsible person and the use of a dosette box or blister pack is recommended.

Drug Treatments

Most of the drug treatments for dementia were designed to treat AD, though some patients whose dementia has a vascular element may benefit from their use too.

Cholinesterase Inhibitors

People with AD and DLB are likely to benefit from the prescription of a cholinesterase inhibitor though not all will be helped and some are unable to tolerate the drugs. In many, but not all, developed countries, the cost of these medications is subsidised by insurance schemes or direct government support. The three medications currently in use are donepezil, galantamine and rivastigmine. There is no convincing evidence that any one of these drugs is superior in efficacy to the other two, though there is some suggestion from trials that the latter two may be less well tolerated than donepezil at the upper end of their dosage range. In practice, the choice of drug may hinge upon the mode of administration (see later in the chapter), the dosage schedule or the prescribing practitioner's experience.

All cholinesterase inhibitors have the potential to produce gastrointestinal side effects, especially anorexia, nausea, vomiting, diarrhoea and abdominal discomfort. They tend to slow heart rhythm and may precipitate heart block in vulnerable individuals. Nightmares sometimes occur when cholinesterase inhibitors are prescribed. Some patients get leg cramps when on these drugs.

Donepezil is available as 5 and 10 mg tablets. It is usually given at night to diminish the likelihood of nausea, but many patients tolerate morning administration well and this may reduce the risk of nightmares. The starting dose is 5 mg daily, increasing to 10 mg daily after four weeks. If the 10 mg dose is not tolerated, reversion to 5 mg per day may still be associated with some benefit.

Galantamine is sold as a slow release capsule given once each day. The initial dose is 8 mg daily for one month and then 16 mg per day, increasing to 24 mg if no improvement is seen or when later deterioration becomes manifest.

Rivastigmine is manufactured in capsules, as a liquid and in the form of a skin patch. The capsules and liquid (the latter useful for those who cannot swallow easily) need to be given at least twice daily, because of the drug's short half-life, but the patch is applied once every 24 hours and left in place until the next one is due. Oral administration commences with 3 mg twice daily and aims to reach 6 mg twice daily after two months with an intervening 4.5 mg twice daily dose, but many patients cannot tolerate 12 mg of oral rivastigmine each day. The patch comes in 4.6 mg, 9.5 mg and 13.3 mg strengths, with the 9.5 mg dose being used after one month on 4.6 mg and the highest dose reserved for those who are declining on 9.5 mg per day. Although the patches avoid peak and trough plasma levels and are associated with fewer gastrointestinal side effects than oral rivastigmine, 5 per cent of patients develop skin reactions, which may render long-term use impossible.

In studies of people with AD, cholinesterase inhibitors produce subtle improvements in cognition and function. Between 30 and 60 minutes of supervisory carer time may be saved each day, MMSE scores may rise by a point or two and the patient may be more alert. An apparent slowing in decline is often seen, equivalent to reversing 3–18 months of deterioration. When the extent of any benefit is unclear, a trial off the drug for two to four weeks may indicate (through noticeable worsening of function or behaviour) that the treatment was giving some benefit, in which case it should be restarted. Cessation of a cholinesterase inhibitor in an AD patient who showed an initial drug response should be considered when the patient is severely impaired and no longer mobile or in a stage where palliative care is indicated. Patients should be reviewed frequently when cholinesterase inhibitors are ceased, as even quite impaired patients often seem worse when the drug is stopped and improve when it is restarted.

DLB patients and some with PDD often show significant improvement when treated with a cholinesterase inhibitor, though less trial evidence is available to support their use in this population than for AD. Improvements seen may include a diminution of psychiatric symptoms, including hallucinations, as well as improvement in cognition, and may reflect the fact that the reticular activating system is cholinergically driven and is dysfunctional in both DLB and PDD.

Memantine

Memantine is an N-methyl-d-aspartate (NMDA) receptor antagonist that regulates calcium flux across membranes and may protect against neuronal death. Trials suggest that it has modest efficacy in retarding the progression of moderate to severe AD and may be helpful in mild AD and some forms of VaD. It is usually well tolerated and the standard dose is 20 mg daily (the manufacturer advises a starting dose of 5 mg daily, building up to 20 mg over three to four weeks). Its use may be considered in AD patients with moderate impairments who do not tolerate a cholinesterase inhibitor, or concomitantly with a cholinesterase inhibitor when AD patients are deteriorating despite being on a cholinesterase inhibitor. Memantine is subsidised in fewer places than are the cholinesterase inhibitor drugs, and in some countries it is not possible to have both types of drugs subsidised simultaneously for the same patient.

Drug Treatment of VaD

The first consideration in dementia secondary to vascular disease is to ensure that vascular risk factors, particularly hypertension, are optimally managed. Where atrial fibrillation is present, anti-arrhythmics and anticoagulants may be used. Some trial evidence supports the use of cholinesterase inhibitors and/or memantine in patients with VaD though the margin of benefit is small at best and typically less than that seen in AD or LBD/PDD.

Other Drugs

The use of psychotropic drugs in people with dementia will be addressed in Chapter 5.

A large number of putative disease-modifying treatments for AD have been evaluated in trials. Most focus on one or more elements of the amyloid cascade. Results have been disappointing. While it is possible that disease-modifying treatments for AD will become available eventually, the greatest potential for such treatments may be in the prophylactic treatment of overtly healthy people at high risk of developing symptomatic AD in future (i.e. those with preclinical AD).

Social Management

Referral to a local Alzheimer's association or society for education and advice should be offered to all newly diagnosed dementia patients and their carers. Driving should be assessed if the person with dementia wants to keep driving. If the patient is competent to cede EPOA and make any changes to an existing will or draft a new one, these things should be done soon after diagnosis.

A wide variety of community supports, such as day centres, in-home respite, home help, bathing attendants, visiting nurses and carer support groups, is available in most developed countries and their use should be discussed with patients and families at the start of the illness and at routine follow-up visits thereafter.

The utilisation of residential care for people with dementia varies markedly around the globe. The best care homes have activity programmes for residents and sufficient trained staff to attend to their needs, including psychological as well as physical needs. Psychiatric consultation with residential care facilities by multidisciplinary teams that work closely with GPs, nurses and allied health staff in such settings offers potential benefits to residents and staff.

Carer Support

Family carers of dementia patients experience much higher levels of burden, stress and distress than age-matched members of the general population. Considerable research evidence indicates that many of the adverse consequences of caring can be minimised by education, support and intervention, especially when this assistance commences at an early stage of the dementia. Therefore, in dementia care, the focus should be on the dyad of the person with dementia and their main carer. Timely medical, psychological and practical support matched to the needs of the patient and their carer should be planned and implemented early to anticipate, forestall and manage the stresses and strains that accompany caring for a person with dementia. In most countries, contact with the local Alzheimer's or dementia association offers an ideal starting point for access to education, information and carer support.

Outcome

It has been said that life is a sexually transmitted fatal disease. People with dementia die eventually, as everyone does. They die excessively in accidents and of pneumonia. Quality of life in mild and even moderate dementia is often good, but suffering and distress are more common in the later stages of the syndrome. In advanced dementia, the utility of medical treatment of incident illness needs to be balanced against the likelihood of producing any meaningful improvement in quality of life and the long-term prognosis of the illness. Studies investigating survival in late onset dementia report survival of about six years from diagnosis. Increased severity of cognition and function are risk factors for earlier death. Getting clear information about the patient's views on life-prolonging treatments at an early stage of the dementia can inform practice when dementia is advanced, and families should be closely involved in decisions about end-of-life care. Preparation of an advanced care directive is strongly advised.

Conclusion

Since World War II, there have been remarkable advances in our understanding of dementia and our management of the syndrome. People with dementia and their carers should have the right to receive care informed by accumulated knowledge, and as a consequence, the experience of dementia should be better for current and future generations than for past ones. With the current rapid and sustained increase in biological, clinical and social research into the dementias, a bright light can at last be seen shining at the end of the dementia tunnel.

Further Reading

Articles

Ames, D. *et al.* (2008). For debate: is the evidence for the efficacy of cholinesterase inhibitors in the symptomatic treatment of Alzheimer's disease convincing or not? *International Psychogeriatrics*, 20, 259–292.

The final word(s) on the controversy about the utility of cholinesterase inhibitors to treat AD?

Clarfield, A. M. (2003). The decreasing prevalence of reversible dementias: an updated meta-analysis. *Archives of Internal Medicine*, 163, 2219–2229.

An excellent summary of the evidence in relation to the nature and prevalence of so-called reversible dementias.

Livingston, G. *et al.* (2017). Dementia prevention, intervention and care (The *Lancet* Commission on dementia). *The Lancet*, 390, 10113. doi: 10.1016/S0140-6736(17)31363-6.

Livingston, G. *et al.* (2020). Dementia prevention, intervention, and care: 2020 report of the Lancet Commission. *The Lancet*, 396, 413–446. doi: 10.1016/S0140-6736(20)30367-6.

The two Lancet Commission reports provide clear comprehensive summaries of available evidence about the epidemiology, prevention, treatment and care of dementia.

Journal Supplement

Almeida, O., Flicker, L. and Lautenschlager, N. L. (Guest editors) (2005). Uncommon dementias. *International Psychogeriatrics*, 17 (Supp.1) S79–S92.

Very comprehensive and detailed coverage of the less common but nevertheless important types of dementia, including early onset dementias.

Books

Ames, D., O'Brien, J. T. and Burns, A. (eds.) (2017). *Dementia, 5th ed.* Boca Raton, FL: CRC Press, 916 pp.

An encyclopaedic 900-page compilation of information about all aspects of dementia.

Burns, A. and Waldemar, G. (2017). *Alzheimer's Disease*, 2nd ed. Oxford: Oxford University Press.

A brief but comprehensive overview of the commonest form of dementia.

Evans, S., Garner, J. and Darnley-Smith, R. (eds.) (2020). *Psychodynamic Approaches to the Experience of Dementia: Perspectives from Observation, Theory and Practice*. London: Routledge.

A recent discussion of psychodynamic perspectives on dementia.

Behavioural and Psychological Symptoms of Dementia

Introduction

In addition to her cognitive difficulties, Alzheimer's original patient, Augusta D, exhibited agitation, paranoid delusions and mood symptoms, which were the main reasons for her admission to hospital, and it is far more common for behavioural symptoms rather than cognitive decline to prompt entry to long-term care.

Systematic study of what variously have been termed the non-cognitive, neuropsychiatric, behavioural and psychological, or behavioural and psychiatric symptoms of dementia dates back to the mid-1980s at the earliest, and it is only since then that robust scales for rating these phenomena have emerged. Consequently, descriptive and intervention studies have proliferated over the last three decades.

The term Behavioural and Psychological Symptoms of Dementia (BPSD) arose from a consensus conference organised by the International Psychogeriatric Association (IPA). The varied and diffuse nature of the symptoms grouped under this heading (see Table 5.1) limits the utility of the term, but its promulgation has done much to draw attention to this heterogeneous and important collection of phenomena.

Specific Symptoms

Table 5.1 lists common BPSD symptoms exhibited by people with dementia. Over 60 per cent of older people living in the community with dementia are reported by relatives to exhibit one or more of these symptoms at any time, and in half of these cases the symptom is at least of moderate intensity, while over 90 per cent of people with dementia will experience at least one BPSD that needs specific management at some point in their illness. However, while it is common for individuals with dementia to exhibit such symptoms, these phenomena tend to wax and wane over time, certain symptoms are characteristic of certain stages of the dementia syndrome and some symptoms (e.g. visual hallucinations in dementia with Lewy bodies) are more common in some dementias than in others.

BPSD is an umbrella term. People with dementia who exhibit BPSD have in common the fact that they have a dementia and experience symptoms or behaviours which trouble either themselves or those around them. However, the diffuse nature of BPSD implies that every patient needs an individualised assessment and that the management strategy for one type of BPSD symptom usually will be very different to that required for another type or group of symptoms.

Table 5.1 Behavioural and psychological symptoms of dementia

Mood symptoms
Depression
Anxiety
Euphoria
Apathy

Psychotic symptoms
Delusions
Hallucinations
Misidentifications

Vegetative disorders
Sleep–wake cycle disturbances
Disorders of motor behaviour
Sexual disinhibition or aggression

Other phenomena
Resistance to care interventions
Unprovoked physical or verbal aggression
Disruptive vocalisation (noisy behaviour)

Note: Treatment should be targeted to the relief of specific symptoms.

Natural History of BPSD

Symptoms of depression and anxiety are common in the premonitory stages of dementia before a diagnosis has been made, as well as in patients with mild to moderate dementia. While it is not uncommon for anxiety symptoms to be present at later stages of dementia, depressive symptoms tend to be less common in advanced dementia, though such symptoms are harder to assess in a severely demented individual in whom assessment of mood by traditional mental state examination will be rendered difficult by comprehensive and expressive language difficulties.

Delusions and hallucinations are uncommon in very mild Alzheimer's or vascular dementia, but become more common as dementia advances. Misidentifications of formerly familiar people and places can lead to marked agitation as individuals seek to leave their homes to find some former residence or reject individual family members whom they no longer recognise. As is the case with depressive symptoms, patients with very advanced dementia rarely manifest clear-cut hallucinatory or delusional phenomena, but again, eliciting a description of such experiences from a person with severe dementia may be all but impossible.

A common reason for a psychiatrist to be asked to assess a person with dementia living in residential care is because of resistance to care interventions or aggressive behaviour directed towards other residents or staff. Although such resistive behaviour tends to be due to an inability to comprehend the need for or the nature of care interventions, the progressive loss of physical condition and mobility that accompany the dementia syndrome in its advanced stages often render such aggressive and resistive behaviour less problematic.

Apathy is particularly common in advanced dementia.

Assessment of the Patient with Possible BPSD

It is essential to ask both patients and carers (these may be family members or professional staff) about BPSD symptoms whenever a patient with a dementia is assessed for the first time or reviewed in routine follow-up. The emergence of troublesome BPSDs often acts as a trigger for referral of a patient with dementia to psychiatric services.

The usual routine of history (both from patient and key informants), mental state examination (including an examination of cognitive function), physical examination and targeted special investigations should be followed (in females, a midstream urine specimen will quite often reveal some degree of infection). Among the key questions that need to be addressed are:

- What symptoms are exhibited?
- When, where and in what circumstances are these symptoms manifest?
- Who (if anybody) is troubled by these symptoms and why?
- What management strategies have been tried to date and how effective have they been?

Several instruments have been developed to assess aspects of BPSD. Among the most popular are the Neuropsychiatric Inventory (NPI) and the Cohen Mansfield Agitation Inventory (CMAI).

It is common for treatable physical conditions to exacerbate or cause certain BPSDs, and sometimes drug treatment of these can make the problem worse. For example, severe constipation can lead to distress and agitation, but some antipsychotic or antidepressant medications can cause or worsen constipation. Pain from an arthritic hip or discomfort from a urinary tract infection can be effectively managed without recourse to powerful psychotropic drugs.

Management Principles

The Latin phrase *primum non nocere* (first do no harm) is nowhere more applicable than in the management of individuals with BPSD. Although there is increasing evidence for the utility of certain psychosocial interventions, and some psychotropic drugs have been subject to reasonably rigorous evaluation, it is still fair to say that most interventions lack a large body of robust evidence to support their use and that even where that evidence has been collected, some treatments, especially those that involve drugs, carry with them a significant risk of adverse effects, some of which can be disabling or, very rarely, fatal. Finally, the protean nature of BPSD means that any 'one-size-fits-all' approach is likely to be ineffective or lead to unwanted effects in many cases. It is important to tailor treatment to the symptoms of the individual patient, targeting a specific symptom that may then be monitored to measure success or a need to adjust the therapeutic approach.

In general, once treatable medical causes for BPSD have been eliminated or addressed with appropriate therapies, the standard approach to treatment is to try psychosocial or other non-pharmacological interventions first, followed by a cautious introduction of psychotropic drug monotherapy in cases where there is some evidence of possible efficacy. There may be certain instances where the severity of symptoms warrant immediate introduction of medication targeting the symptom associated with the greatest distress or risk.

Non-pharmacological Management

The systematic evaluation of psychosocial interventions is challenging, given the need to standardise interventions for evaluation by randomised controlled trials using validated outcome measures. Indeed, an expert in this field once wrote that research into the non-pharmacological management of dementia was characterised by unsupported assertions and unreplicated results. Things have improved since these words were written, but it is true that most outcome data from psychosocial intervention studies are characterised by sub-optimal sample sizes, that some studies employ less than robust outcome measures and that a number of approaches which show promising potential have not been subject to rigorous, replicated, randomised controlled trials.

Six basic approaches to treatment can be characterised.

1. Person-centred and family-centred approaches emphasise the need to understand the life history and sociocultural background of the person with dementia and their significant others. This may make some of the patient's behaviours more understandable for staff and lead to more appropriate management. One example of such an approach is the case of a former wool-classer who spent much of the day disrupting bed coverings and shaking them out, as he would have done with wool fleeces years earlier. When he was given a pile of blankets, a table and a room to shake them in, staff of the residential facility where he lived found his behaviour to be better contained and easier to deal with.

2. Caring for carers emphasises the fact that carers have needs for self-fulfilment and activity which in most cases are not entirely met by caring for their demented relative, even where this is not explicitly admitted or acknowledged. Carer burnout, depression and anxiety are common and can lead to both the patient and the carer experiencing deterioration in health and well-being. A number of evidence-based approaches focus on caring for carers. Respite care, increased home support and carer support groups may help to address some of these needs and make it easier for a tired or overwhelmed carer to continue the caring role.

3. Randomised controlled trials indicate that training formal and informal carers in how to manage behavioural symptoms may reduce carer burnout and reduce BPSD. For example, carer training groups or nurse practitioners using a collaborative care model may offer effective help in the management of BPSD.

4. Community outreach, again focused on the provision of assistance and advice provided by nurses, also has supportive trial evidence.

5. The utilisation of implicit memory (i.e. that which is recalled unconsciously and without effort) has been the subject of one nurse-centred RCT and shows promise.

6. Finally, the use of non-contingent positive regard (be nice to people and they are more likely to be nice to you) has anecdotal and some trial evidence for its utility.

These six approaches can be boiled down to three major avenues of assistance. One is to utilise behaviour management techniques to diminish the frequency of undesirable behaviours through positive reinforcement of desirable ones. The second is to train and empower both family and professional carers through education, and thereby to enhance their management skills, and thus to diminish the negative consequences (burden, stress, anxiety, depression) of caring. A third approach is the utilisation of specific interventions for specific behaviours. The simulated presence of a significant other (often through tape recording of voice) is reported to be effective in diminishing both physical and verbal agitation. The use of music, individually matched to the past preferences of the individual receiving therapy, or which is associated with meaningful memories, appears helpful in diminishing physical agitation. Structured physical activity improved competence in activities of daily living but may not always diminish the frequency or intensity of behaviours of concern. Finally, aromatherapy, while popular, has only modest evidence to support its use in the amelioration of BPSD (lavender oil is the agent that has been most studied).

Pharmacological Management

Table 5.2 lists a large number of drug treatments, all of which have two things in common. First, all of these drugs have at some time been used or advocated for use in treating or controlling certain BPSD. Second, none of these drugs was developed for the specific purpose of treating individuals with dementia for disturbed behaviour or psychological symptoms. Therefore, it is not surprising that these treatments do not always 'work' when given to behaviourally disturbed or psychologically distressed individuals affected by dementia.

Antipsychotic Drugs

Reasonable evidence exists to suggest that some novel antipsychotic drugs, particularly low-dose risperidone in doses between 0.5 and 2 mg daily (use of risperidone for this purpose has been better studied than is the case for any other drug), may have modest efficacy in ameliorating psychosis, aggression and agitation. The effect is not mediated solely by the induction of somnolence, and while the evidence is best for risperidone, there are some positive results for the use of olanzapine, aripiprazole and brexpiprazole for this indication. No other novel antipsychotic has evidence of efficacy in this regard. Evidence for the older classical antipsychotic drugs, such as haloperidol, is weaker as most of the few, small trials of these drugs took place before the development of modern instruments for the evaluation of efficacy.

Unfortunately, there is strong evidence that classical antipsychotics commonly cause troublesome extrapyramidal side effects in people with dementia, that they may exacerbate Parkinsonism and may occasionally be associated with fatal adverse events when used to treat people with DLB. Use of the atypical antipsychotics risperidone and olanzapine in

Table 5.2 Drugs that have been used or advocated for the treatment of BPSD: few have clear efficacy and many have significant adverse effects

Novel antipsychotics
Classical antipsychotics
Antidepressants
Benzodiazepines
Lithium
Anticonvulsants (valproate, carbemazepine)
Barbiturates
Cholinesterase inhibitors
Oestrogen
Cyproterone acetate

people with dementia is associated with threefold increase in the risk of (both serious and non-serious) cerebrovascular adverse events (CVAEs) and there is some evidence to suggest that this risk is at least as high, if not higher, when classical antipsychotics are used for the same indication. The mechanism by which the risk of such CVAEs is raised remains obscure, but effects on blood pressure and coagulability do not seem to explain the risk. Individuals with poorly controlled cardiac arrhythmias, hypertension, diabetes and previous stroke were very much over-represented in the group experiencing CVAEs in trials, and it is likely that the risk will be substantially lower in dementia patients who do not exhibit these risk factors.

Antidepressants

Trials of antidepressants for the treatment of both depression and agitation in dementia have been small in size and disappointing in results. Citalopram reduced agitation in one trial, though this took several weeks. The best and largest such trial found that neither sertraline nor mirtazapine was any better than placebo at treating depressive symptoms in dementia (though mirtazapine did help anxiety and sleep disturbance), and the recommendation of the Lancet Commission on Dementia is to avoid antidepressants in people with dementia who are depressed, unless there is a previous history of depression or if psychosocial and support measures have failed to help. Tricyclic antidepressants are likely to produce anticholinergic side effects and should not be used to treat depression (or anything else) in most people with dementia, as their central cholinergic systems are likely to be malfunctioning already, without the addition of an anticholinergic drug.

Other Psychotropic Drugs

Cholinesterase inhibitors have a detectable but weak effect in delaying the emergence of BPSD in individuals with AD who start treatment when in the mild stage of dementia. Any evidence that such drugs are effective in treating prevalent agitation or other BPSD symptoms in individuals with more severe dementia is lacking or at best extremely weak. In other words, early treatment with these drugs may help retard the emergence of BPSD in addition to any other benefits on cognition, activity or carer time required for supervision and assistance, but they are not first choice therapy for any element of BPSD in more advanced AD. In DLB, there is evidence from one RCT that rivastigmine may have significant benefit in ameliorating hallucinations, delusions and agitation and the same is true for Parkinson's disease dementia.

Despite advocacy for their use made on the basis of early small studies, most trials of anticonvulsants in the management of BPSD have met with limited or no success (these trials have focused upon the use of sodium valproate and carbamazepine, but negative trials of gabapentin, lamotrigine and topiramate also have been reported). A 2008 review of the literature concluded that there was no convincing basis upon which to advocate their routine use, though more recent work with carbamazepine has suggested some possible limited benefit.

In summary, antidepressants should be used in dementia when other measures have failed or there is convincing history of previous depression responding to treatment before dementia developed. Where aggression or psychosis is prominent, low-dose risperidone (0.5–2 mg daily) is the drug of choice, with olanzapine (2.5–10 mg daily) as second line therapy if extrapyramidal side effects prove problematic. Aripiprazole also may be useful. Patients' relatives should be informed of the increased risk of CVAEs and other possible side effects associated with such therapy. Excluding individuals at high risk of stroke may diminish the incidence of CVAEs. Cholinesterase inhibitors may delay the emergence of BPSD in some people with AD but are of little benefit except for symptoms of DLB or PDD.

Conclusions

In no area of old age psychiatry is the need for more research on effective safe therapies, which show reasonable efficacy, more pressing than in the area of BPSD. Current best practice should involve a thorough assessment of individuals with dementia who exhibit aggressive or distressing behaviours or dysphoric psychological symptoms, an optimal management of any underlying or comorbid medical problems, evaluation and manipulation of environmental precipitants, education of both professional and family carers, use of some specific behavioural interventions in some cases and cautious use of antidepressants or novel antipsychotics where specifically indicated for individual symptoms of moderate or greater severity.

Further Reading

Articles

Ames, D. et al. (2005). For debate: should novel antipsychotics ever be used to treat the behavioral and psychological symptoms of dementia (BPSD)? *International Psychogeriatrics*, 17, 3–29. doi: 10.1017/S104161020521102-X.

This article summarises the pros and cons of using antipsychotics to treat BPSD.

Brodaty, H. et al. (2003). A randomized placebo controlled trial of Risperidone for the treatment of agitation and psychosis of dementia. *Journal of Clinical Psychiatry*, 64, 134–143. doi: 10.4088/jcp.v64n0205.

A good example of a well-conducted drug trial, this paper illustrates the challenges of conducting such studies as well as highlighting both beneficial and adverse effects of therapy.

Cohen Mansfield, J., Marx, M. S. and Rosenthal, A. S. (1989). A description of agitation in a nursing home. *Journal of Gerontology*, 44, M77–M84. doi: 10.1093/geronj/44.3.m77.

This paper contains a description of the Cohen-Mansfield Agitation Inventory, one of the most widely used and useful scales in the assessment of BPSD.

Cummings, J. L. et al. (1994). The Neuropsychiatric Inventory: comprehensive assessment of psychopathology in dementia. *Neurology*, 44, 2308–2314. doi: 10.1212/wnl.44.12.2308.

The most popular scale for the assessment of BPSD in research settings.

Konovalov, S., Murali, S. and Tampi, R. R. (2008). Anticonvulsants for the treatment of behavioral and psychological symptoms of dementia: a literature review. *International Psychogeriatrics*, 20, 293–308. doi: 10/1017/S1041610207006540.

This review concludes that there is little evidence to support the use of anticonvulsants to treat BPSD.

Livingston, G. et al. (2017). Dementia prevention, intervention and care (The Lancet Commission on dementia). *The Lancet*, 390, 10113. doi: 10.1016/S0140-6736(17) 31363–6.

Livingston, G. et al. (2020). Dementia prevention, intervention, and care: 2020 report of the Lancet Commission. *The Lancet*, 396, 413–446. doi: 10.1016/S0140-6736(20)30367-6.

The two Lancet Commission reports provide clear comprehensive summaries of available evidence about the epidemiology, prevention, treatment and care of dementia, including BPSD/neuropsychiatric symptoms.

Books

Ames, D., Burns, A and O'Brien J. T. (2017). *Dementia, 4th ed.* London: CRC Press.

This comprehensive textbook covers virtually all aspects of dementia and has good chapters on the assessment and management of BPSD, including psychosocial and pharmacological approaches.

Moulds, R. *et al.* (2013). *Therapeutic Guidelines Psychotropic Version 7.* Melbourne: Therapeutic Guidelines.

An excellent guide to the utilisation of psychopharmacological strategies in all forms of mental illness, including dementia.

Delirium

Introduction

Delirium in old age is common, clinically important, costly and potentially preventable. It is the most frequent complication following hospital admission in late life, and is often due to a failure of care. Health professionals sometimes lack the necessary knowledge, skills and attitudes to assess, manage and prevent delirium in the modern high-technology, fast-throughput hospital environment, and the result is adverse outcomes for patients and a huge waste of resources. Interventions can reduce the incidence of hospital-acquired delirium and limit its impact should it occur.

Clinical Features

Delirium was one of the first mental disorders to be identified; recognisable descriptions of transient derangements of mental functioning due to illness, injury and intoxication can be found in the ancient Greek Hippocratic texts. The subsequent history of the concept is complex and confusing, but the following have consistently been recognised as core features: disturbance of consciousness, disturbance of thinking (cognition), rapid onset, fluctuating course and evidence of some external cause. It is an acute disorder, and usually resolves with treatment of the underlying causes, but the long-term outcomes for older patients are often poor.

There are no diagnostic tests for delirium. Making the diagnosis depends upon a careful assessment of its clinical characteristics. The key differential diagnoses are other causes of cognitive impairment, notably dementia in elderly patients, but this distinction is complicated by the fact that dementia is an important risk factor for delirium, and often underlies it. A history of rapid onset (within days) and fluctuating course of cognitive impairment is strongly indicative of a delirium, but the patient will usually not be in a position to describe this, and a history from family, care staff or nursing records is essential. In some instances, the onset of a delirium can be more insidious, for example, the slow accumulation of drugs, but even here the development is over weeks rather than the months or years that are more typical for a dementia.

Delirium is not an all-or-nothing phenomenon, and a full-blown episode meeting formal diagnostic criteria is usually preceded by a prodromal phase as the disorder develops. In some cases, the delirium may resolve before the full syndrome manifests, and never achieve diagnostic status. In this prodrome, the patient may be able to cooperate with formal mental state assessment and will describe feeling muddled and unable to concentrate. Perceptions of time and space are distorted, and it takes effort to keep a grip on reality. The sleep–wake cycle is often disturbed in the early stages, with sleep during the day and alertness at night, and patients may feel either irritable or lethargic. As the delirium develops, the disturbance of consciousness leads to progressively reduced awareness of the external environment, and reduction of the ability to focus, sustain and shift attention; this attentional deficit quickly alerts experienced clinicians to the possibility of the diagnosis. Cognitive impairments in delirium include disorientation in time and place, memory deficits and language disturbances. Sensory perception, both visual and auditory, may be disturbed, resulting in misinterpretations, illusions and hallucinations. Patients interviewed about their experiences following an episode of delirium describe an awareness of their confused state, and how they struggle to regain control and understanding of their situation. The acute mental disturbances of delirium are often very frightening and distressing for patients, who may respond with agitated and aggressive behaviour. If the delirium is severe, or if there is significant accompanying dementia, formal mental state assessment may not be possible, and the delirium will need to be inferred from the effects it has on behaviour and other aspects of functioning, such as mobility, continence and activities of daily living (ADL).

One of the diagnostic problems with delirium is that it can manifest itself in a hyperactive form, in a hypoactive form or in a combination or alteration between these states. The exemplar for the hyperactive form of delirium is the acute alcohol withdrawal state known as *delirium tremens*; the patient is aroused and irritable, and often angry, fearful and aggressive in response to hallucinations in a range of modalities. There may be autonomic arousal and neurological symptoms such as tremor and myoclonus. By contrast, in hypoactive delirium there is drowsiness, apparent apathy and underactivity, with slowing of thought, speech and movement. Hyperactive delirium is more often seen in younger adults, and perhaps for this reason has tended to dominate the historical descriptions that underpin perceptions of and criteria for the disorder. It is clinically conspicuous, and its detection and diagnosis is relatively straightforward. By contrast, the hypoactive delirium that is seen more often in older adults is much less obvious, particularly if there is a pre-existing dementia. As a result, it is quite common for delirium in an elderly patient to be overlooked by medical and nursing staff – in up to 95 per cent of cases in some studies.

Improving the recognition of delirium is a prerequisite to its effective management, and nurses may be in a better position to do this than doctors, as they are in contact with patients for longer periods of time and can observe fluctuations in the mental state. However, this information needs to be communicated to all members of the clinical team if it is to be useful. Routine, repeated assessment of cognitive function is important, particularly in those patients identified as being at risk of developing delirium. A number of instruments, such as the Confusion Assessment Method (CAM), the Delirium Rating Scale (DRS) and the 4AT (www.the4AT.com), have been developed to assist with the detection and monitoring of delirium, but a simple brief cognitive screen, such as the Mini-mental State Examination (MMSE) or clock drawing, while not diagnostic, can also be useful to identify cognitive decline, and may be more practical in non-psychiatric settings.

Differential Diagnosis

Delirium can mimic most of the organic and functional mental disorders that occur in old age. Like dementia, conditions such as depression, mania and schizophrenia in old age can also predispose to delirium, either through self-neglect or exhaustion or because of the powerful psychotropic drugs used to treat them, so the possibility of comorbidity must be considered. Delirium, like fever or pain, is an important non-specific sign that a patient is physically ill; if the diagnosis is in doubt, investigate as if it were a delirium.

Delirium and Dementia

In principle, this is an important differential diagnosis to consider, because of the dire consequences of misdiagnosis. In practice, since dementia is the most important vulnerability factor for delirium in elderly patients (see the section Risk Factors later in the chapter), comorbidity is common. Indeed, the appearance of delirium in an apparently cognitively intact elderly individual should prompt a careful assessment for the early signs of dementia once the patient has recovered, since this may be the first sign that the patient is becoming vulnerable in this respect. However, there are pitfalls for the unwary. Faced with a delirious patient, clinicians often become impatient if physical recovery is not quickly followed by cognitive recovery, and if the patient remains cognitively impaired for any length of time, this may be attributed to dementia and the patient managed accordingly. In fact, delirium can be quite persistent in old age, so there is a risk that important life-changing interventions, such as admission to a nursing home, may be made while there is still potential for further cognitive and functional improvement. It has been suggested that delirium and dementia may be related at a more fundamental pathophysiological level, as different manifestations of various acute and chronic inflammatory processes in the brain (see section Neuropathophysiology later in the chapter).

Delirium and Mood Disorders

Depression is another important differential diagnosis of delirium in elderly patients, particularly those with dementia. Like delirium, depression can present with cognitive and functional decline, and disturbances in behaviour and sleep. Diurnal variation in mood may be mistaken for the fluctuations of a delirium, although typically, delirious patients are better in the early part of the day, unlike those with depression. Depression tends to develop more slowly, but within the timescale of a subacute delirium. A previous history of episodes of either depression or delirium may be helpful, particularly if the clinical features have been documented.

While depression in old age can sometimes resemble hypoactive delirium, mania is often mistaken for hyperactive delirium. If the patient has a long history of bipolar disorder, the differential diagnosis is not usually problematic, but mania can occur for the first time in old age, often in association with organic cerebral pathology. In all cases, comorbid delirium is quite common, due to exhaustion and self-neglect.

Neuropathophysiology

The pathogenesis of delirium is not well understood, but many of the functional cortical and sub-cortical areas of the brain are involved, particularly the association cortices, the limbic system and the ascending cholinergic and monoaminergic systems. Electroencephalography (EEG) and evoked potentials show diffuse slowing, and single photon emission computed tomography (SPECT) and positron emission tomography (PET) studies show abnormalities across many brain regions. However, despite this extensive neuronal derangement in response to a wide range of toxic, metabolic and traumatic causes, the relatively limited and stereotyped nature of the core syndrome suggests that there may be a final common pathway for delirium.

There is some evidence for both the structural (neuroanatomical) and functional (neurophysiological) aspects of this pathway. Studies of delirium following stroke suggest it is more common after right-sided (non-dominant) lesions, particularly those involving the posterior parietal cortex and thalamus. At the functional level, there is a growing body of evidence that the delirium is the result of an imbalance in cholinergic and dopaminergic neurotransmission (reduced cholinergic/excess dopaminergic). Muscarinic cholinergic neurotransmission is involved in many of the brain functions that are deranged in delirium: cortical arousal, maintenance of EEG fast wave activity, REM sleep, memory and learning, maintaining attention and motor activity. Anticholinergic drugs are particularly prone to induce delirium, especially in those whose cholinergic function is already compromised, such as patients with Alzheimer's disease (AD). This drug-induced delirium can be reversed with cholinesterase inhibitor drugs, such as physostigmine or rivastigmine. Most anticholinergic drugs act as post-synaptic antagonists, although some may influence cholinergic neurotransmission via pre-synaptic receptors, or more indirectly by influencing other modulating neurones. A number of other causes of delirium, such as hypoxia, hyperglycaemia, thiamine deficiency, liver failure and physical damage, also affect cholinergic neurotransmission by reducing acetylcholine (Ach) synthesis; one of the immediate metabolic precursors of Ach is acetyl-co-enzyme A, an important and potentially rate-limiting component of the cellular aerobic citric acid cycle. In many parts of the brain, there is a reciprocal interaction between the cholinergic and dopaminergic systems, with increased dopamine activity resulting from reduced cholinergic activity, and vice versa. Therefore, delirium can be caused by dopamine agonist drugs (e.g. levodopa, bupropion). There is a wide range of dopamine receptor subtypes in the brain, all subserving different functions, and it has been suggested that individual differences in the responsiveness of these, or their differential involvement in different delirium aetiologies, may explain why some delirium is hypoactive (D3 predominant) or hyperactive (D1 predominant). It may be that age-associated changes to the cholinergic and dopaminergic systems, such as reductions in receptor density and plasticity, contribute increased vulnerability to delirium.

While the cholinergic and dopaminergic systems appear to be the most closely involved in the pathophysiology of delirium, others such as the serotonergic and glutamatergic systems are probably also contributory, either by influence upon the cholinergic/dopaminergic neurones or in their own right. Delirium is associated with states of both serotonergic excess (e.g. drug-induced 'serotonin syndrome') and insufficiency (e.g. alcohol withdrawal). Some conditions, such as hypoxia, give rise to surges of toxic neurotransmitters (e.g. glutamate) that may be deliriogenic.

How do severe systemic illness, infection and trauma act on the brain to produce delirium? These conditions activate the immune system and stimulate the production of cytokines. One function of these small polypeptides is to communicate with the CNS to elicit 'sickness behaviour' (reduced activity, appetite, social interaction etc.). They also activate the HPA and HPG axes, alter blood-brain barrier permeability, interfere with cerebral neurotransmission and reduce the activity of neuroprotective cytokines, any or all of which may contribute to delirium in vulnerable individuals. In young adults, this cytokine signalling is self-limiting without any lasting consequences, but conditions such as AD, with a chronic inflammatory component to their pathophysiology, may be accelerated by this process, resulting in more rapid cognitive and functional decline. This may account for the evidence of an association between delirium and subsequent cognitive decline in aged patients.

Epidemiology

There have been many investigations of the prevalence and incidence of delirium in older medical and surgical in-patients, with a wide range of rates reported. There are a number of reasons for this variation: different case definitions, with more or less strict inclusion criteria; different case-finding procedures, from passive methods, such as case note review, to more active strategies, such as patient interview on one or more occasions, which produce a higher yield; and selection bias, including exclusion of the more severely ill and high-risk patients. The variability of prevalence and incidence rates is highest in the earlier, less standardised surveys. More recent studies suggest prevalence rates of 10–20 per cent, and post-admission incidence rates of 5–10 per cent. Some of the variation probably is due to the greater vulnerability of some patient groups, for example older patients following surgery for hip fracture appear to be at particular risk of developing delirium. These figures translate into a significant burden for health services; it has been estimated that in the United States delirium complicates the hospital admission of over 2.3 million people per year, involving over 17.5 million in-patient days at a cost of over $US7 billion (2021 prices). Delirium in other settings has been less extensively studied. One particularly vulnerable group is the frail older population living in nursing homes; some Scandinavian studies have suggested that the prevalence in this setting may be as high as 60 per cent, which raises important questions about the quality of care provided.

Risk Factors

At any age, delirium is the consequence of an interaction between intrinsic vulnerability (predisposing causes) and external insults that affect brain functioning (precipitating causes). In childhood, the principal predisposing cause is the incomplete myelination of the central nervous system. In older adults, neurodegenerative disorders such as dementia are the most important predisposing risk factor for delirium, with an associated relative risk of 5.2 (see section Delirium and Dementia earlier in this chapter). Other predisposing vulnerability factors in this age group include impairments in vision and hearing, which approximately double the risk of developing delirium, if present. Physical illness factors that increase the risk of delirium include severity, instability, comorbidity, functional impairment, malnutrition and dehydration. It is not clear to what extent age itself is a risk factor for delirium, independent of age-associated conditions such as dementia and sensory impairment. Age-related changes in receptor populations, drug binding and metabolism may confer increased vulnerability to this particular cause of delirium; for example, hypoalbuminaemia, which increases the amount of free drug in the plasma, is predictive of delirium. However, elderly individuals vary considerably in these respects. Male sex, alcohol abuse and lower educational attainment have also been identified as predisposing factors for delirium in some studies.

Regarding the precipitating factors, any acute physical illness can cause delirium if the patient is sufficiently vulnerable. Among the commonest causes are infections, metabolic disturbances and conditions that impair oxygen supply to the brain (Table 6.1). Medication is the other common precipitating cause of delirium in elderly patients; again, any drug has the potential to cause delirium, but psychotropic agents, narcotic analgesics, dopamine agonists and drugs with anticholinergic properties have the greatest potential in this respect. Many of the drugs commonly prescribed to elderly patients, such

Table 6.1 Factors precipitating delirium

Medication (prescribed)

Medication (over-the-counter)

Medication (alcohol and illicit drugs)

Infection

Cerebral hypoxia (heart failure, myocardial infarct, stroke etc.)

Metabolic causes

A combination of the above

Something else

Adapted from Rockwood, K. and MacKnight, C. (2001).

as prednisolone, cimetidine and digoxin, have some degree of anticholinergic activity, and it may be the cumulative effect that is important. In more severely demented individuals, urinary retention, faecal impaction and pain may be sufficient to precipitate a delirium, although the mechanisms involved are unclear. Similarly, psychological and environmental disruptions, such as relocation, sleep deprivation, sensory deprivation and bereavement, can contribute to or cause delirium in those who are vulnerable.

The experience of surgery provides the older patient with many opportunities for developing delirium, including pre-operative hypovolaemia and hypothermia, exposure to psychoactive medication (pre-meds, anaesthetics, analgesics) and post-operative sepsis, immobility and sensory deprivation. In fact, modern minimally invasive techniques combined – crucially – with the ability to select 'good-risk' patients means that observed rates of delirium in elective surgical populations are quite low. They are much higher in 'poor-risk' groups where surgery is unavoidable, such as hip-fracture patients.

Several factors related to the process of care increase the risk of developing delirium in hospital, both as predisposing and precipitating causes. These include the number of procedures undergone, bladder catheterisation, polypharmacy, use of physical restraints and malnutrition. Furthermore, most hospital environments and procedures are not designed with cognitively impaired patients in mind, and probably contribute to the development of delirium. These predisposing and precipitating risk factors are highly interrelated and multiplicative in their effect, and a number of predictive models have been developed, in an attempt to identify those patients at particular risk of developing delirium during their hospital stay.

Course and Prognosis

Although usually regarded as a transient disorder, delirium can be prolonged or recurrent in about one-third of elderly patients in hospital; disorientation and memory impairment appear to be particularly slow to recover. Rates of cognitive recovery at hospital discharge range between 40 per cent and 70 per cent. Some groups, such as those admitted from nursing homes, appear to have a particularly poor outcome in this respect. Patients who have been delirious, but not previously known to have dementia, are at increased risk of developing dementia subsequently. This may be because those in the preclinical stages of dementia are more vulnerable to delirium; alternatively, delirium may have persistent neurotoxic effects on the brain. If delirium is shown to contribute to the development of dementia, this will further emphasise the need for primary prevention (see later in the chapter).

Delirium is associated with significant physical ill health or intoxication, so it is not surprising that it is associated with adverse outcomes, such as increased mortality and morbidity, increased length of hospital stay, increased dependency and short- and long-term functional decline and institutionalisation following discharge. However, delirium also impedes the processes of diagnosis, management and rehabilitation, and increases the risk of developing other hospital-acquired complications; hypoactive patients may develop pressure sores and chest and urinary tract infections, and hyperactive patients are at risk from hip fracture following falls. Consequently, there is a significant independent association between delirium and the various categories of adverse outcome that have been studied, which underlines the importance of prompt and effective management of the condition, and prevention where possible.

Management

The evidence base for effective management strategies in delirium is limited. Clinical reviews and practice guidelines identify four key components to the effective management of delirium in the older patient: address the underlying causes; maintain behavioural control; prevent common complications; and rehabilitation.

Address the Underlying Causes

Effective diagnostic assessment of delirium is the starting point for its management. This should focus on the commonest causes: medications, infections, metabolic disorders and conditions causing impaired oxygenation of the CNS (e.g. anaemia, congestive cardiac failure, chronic obstructive pulmonary disease). Any newly started, increased, or recently discontinued medications should be considered, as should the possibility of adverse drug interactions. Remember that alcohol is a drug. Infections in elderly patients are not always obvious, and delirium may be the presenting feature of a chest infection, cellulitis or a urinary tract infection. Dehydration is a common cause of metabolic disruption leading to delirium, particularly in vulnerable groups such as nursing home populations. Other factors that commonly cause or contribute to delirium, such as sensory impairment, constipation and urinary retention and pain, should be identified. A simple cause-and-effect model for delirium in old age is usually inappropriate; any individual case is likely to be the consequence of a number of predisposing and precipitating factors acting together, and all need to be addressed in management. Disruptive and invasive investigations, such as MRI scans or lumbar puncture, are not necessary unless clearly indicated by the clinical history, or if the initial search for common causes is negative.

There are no drugs available that will reverse delirium, although cholinesterase inhibitors have attracted interest in this regard. Delirium secondary to alcohol or sedative withdrawal may be treated with a tapering course of a benzodiazepine such as oxazepam or lorazepam.

Maintain Behavioural Control

Disturbed behaviour is very poorly tolerated in modern in-patient units, and quickly leads to demands for sedation. However, as with disturbed behaviour in dementia, it is important to consider why the patient is distressed and address the underlying cause wherever possible. In the case of delirium, this is usually because the patient is unable to make sense of what they perceive as an alien and hostile environment. The reassuring presence of family members can be very helpful, as can the provision of consistent nursing staff. All interactions with the patient should be calm, non-confrontational and orienting, and interventions should be carefully explained in a step-by-step way. Modifications of hospital environment and routines, including use of non-pharmacological sleep protocols, are effective in restoring normal sleep–wake cycles, but are labour intensive and hard to achieve in most hospital systems.

Sometimes chemical or physical restraint may be necessary to protect the patient or others, but if they are not used with care, they may make the situation worse. Unsupervised physical restraint increases the risk of injury and falls, and excessive or inappropriate psychotropic medication may deepen and prolong the delirium. The limited evidence base in this area favours the use of high potency antipsychotic drugs such as haloperidol; they are probably most effective when the disturbed behaviour is secondary to psychotic symptoms, such as hallucinations. Initially haloperidol should be prescribed at a low dose (0.5–1 mg), with frequent review to titrate changes in the dose against response; the aim should be to give the lowest effective dose for the shortest possible time. Atypical antipsychotic drugs may have a role in patients with Parkinson's disease or dementia with Lewy bodies (DLB), where haloperidol should not be used. Recent evidence suggests that use of benzodiazepines may prolong the duration of delirium, so their use (particularly the use of those with long half lives like diazepam) should be avoided if possible.

Prevent Common Complications

Once the underlying causes of the delirium have been corrected, it may take some time for an elderly patient to regain their previous level of functioning, and they will be vulnerable to a wide range of complications that may lead to enduring functional impairment and even death. A crucial aspect of delirium management is to prevent and manage these complications, the commonest of which are urinary incontinence, immobility, falls, pressure sores, sleep disruption, dehydration and malnutrition. Patients should have a programme of regular toileting (*not* an indwelling catheter), supervised and structured mobilisation and physiotherapy, a sleep hygiene programme, assistance with feeding and careful monitoring of food and fluid intake.

Rehabilitation

As the patient recovers, the focus of management shifts to a programme of rehabilitation aimed at a return to the pre-morbid state of functioning. The level of basic ADL capacity should be assessed regularly, and the patient encouraged to do what they can for themselves wherever possible. The patient's immediate environment should be made as non-threatening and orienting as possible, with regular routines and reminders about the date, time and place. It is important to involve family members in this process: they are an important source of information about pre-morbid functioning; they can contribute to bedside care and support; they have access to familiar and orienting materials, such as photographs; they will have concerns about the cause and the prognosis that will need to be addressed; and they will be heavily involved in the supervision and aftercare of the patient once they have been discharged from hospital. Delirium is often recurrent, and the family should be advised to be alert for the early signs of this. There is very little evidence about the effect of post-discharge rehabilitation and support; one study suggests that a relatively modest package of case management and rehabilitation can significantly reduce the use of long-term institutional care. Delirium may be a useful marker of vulnerability in elderly inpatients, and of the need for more intensive community aftercare than is usually provided for this population.

Prevention

The evidence base is rather better so far as the prevention of delirium is concerned. An understanding of the multiple risk factors for delirium in hospital settings has led to the development of predictive models, and the evaluation of interventions designed to reduce its incidence. In the Yale-New Haven Study, the intervention consisted of a series of management protocols for cognitive impairment, sleep deprivation, immobility, visual impairment, hearing impairment and dehydration. These were carried out by a trained multidisciplinary team supported by volunteers. When compared to care-as-usual, there was a 40 per cent reduction in the incidence of delirium in the intervention group, with patients at intermediate levels of risk obtaining the greatest benefit. Based on this study's findings, this programme has been successfully established in three medical units within a hospital, and it appears to be cost-effective.

Studies of geriatric consultation services to general medical and surgical units have produced mixed results; a key factor appears to be the extent to which the recommendations are adhered to by medical and nursing staff.

There is more scope for preventing delirium in surgical patients, since the immediate cause is usually planned, and there is time for preparing and optimising the patient. A range of interventions is modestly effective in reducing the incidence of delirium in this population, including preoperative chest physiotherapy, explanation, support and anxiety management; peri-operative maintenance of blood pressure and oxygen tension; and post-operative pain management, including patient-controlled analgesia.

A common theme across many intervention strategies is the need to educate health professionals in contact with patients about the importance of delirium, its complications and how to identify and manage it effectively. Occasional and ad hoc training activities are unlikely to be effective on their own; delirium needs to form part of all medical and nursing school curricula, with clearly defined learning aims and outcomes. If training can be linked to formal ward-based delirium prevention programmes, so much the better.

Conclusion

Delirium may be regarded as a marker of the quality of hospital care, in terms of physical design, organisation and management, the awareness and training of medical and nursing staff in the recognition and effective management of the problem and links with community support services. Given the mean age of most medical and surgical inpatient populations in developed societies, there is an urgent need to develop hospital environments, systems of care and clinical teams that are equipped to meet their needs. Achieving this alongside the onward march of medical technology will not be easy; demonstrable cost-effectiveness is probably the key to implementation.

Further Reading

Articles

Cole, M. (2004). Delirium in elderly patients. *American Journal of Psychiatry*, 12, 7–21.

A good overview, which has not dated much.

Inouye, S. K., Schlesinger, M. J. and Lydon, T. J. (1999). Delirium: a symptom of how hospital care is failing older persons and a window to improve quality of hospital care. *American Journal of Medicine*, 106, 563–573. doi: 10.1016/s0002-9343(99)00070-4.

This article, whose first author has done as much as anyone to bring the challenge of delirium to clinical attention, is as pertinent now as when it was published.

Tieges, Z. *et al.* (2020). Diagnostic accuracy of the 4AT for delirium detection: systematic review and meta-analysis. *Age and Ageing*, 50, 733–743. doi: 10.1093/ageing/afaa224.

Diagnostic test accuracy for a new, promising delirium screening instrument.

Wilson, J. E. *et al.* (2020). Delirium. *Nature Reviews Disease Primers* 6, 90. doi: 10.1038/s41572-020-00223-4.

Very up-to-date review.

Book

Rahman, S. (2020). *Essentials of Delirium: Everything You Really Need to Know for Working in Delirium Care*. London: Jessica Kingsley Publishers.

Excellent modern overview endorsed by Sharon Inouye.

Chapter 7

Mood Disorders in Late Life

DEPRESSION

Introduction

The ubiquity of losses in old age might invite the conclusion that depression is an inevitable consequence of living into late life. However, evidence does not support this hypothesis and, hence, one must be vigilant about dismissing depressive symptoms in older adults as inevitable or 'understandable'. The clinical implication is that those patients with persistent depressive symptoms, as defined in this chapter, must be taken seriously and be properly assessed and managed.

Nosology and Classification

The diagnosis of depression is defined in contemporary psychiatry by the classification systems of the International Classification of Diseases (ICD-11) as well as the American Psychiatric Association (DSM-5). Tables 7.1 and 7.2 outline the definitions for both systems of the more commonly diagnosed forms of depression and dysthymia.

Comorbidity

Compared to younger people, older people experience a higher level of comorbidity of medical diseases, including those that cause the syndromes of dementias and mild cognitive impairment. These two features can make depression, particularly late onset depression, a challenge to diagnose and treat.

Cognitive Impairment, Dementia and the Phenomenology of Depression

Notwithstanding the evidence suggesting that late life depression sometimes may be a prodrome of dementia, there is a lot of evidence to suggest that depression represents an independent risk factor predisposing to dementia. This is true even when depressive symptoms occur many years prior to the onset of dementia. Indeed, lifetime history of depression represents a significant increase in the risk of Alzheimer's disease (AD), independent of family history for dementia. Similarly, there is evidence that a history of depression is a risk factor for vascular dementia too.

Several studies have noted a prevalence of 30–50 per cent for depressive symptoms in AD (the most common of the dementias – see Chapter 4). This high prevalence of

Table 7.1 ICD-11 depressive disorders – summary

Depressive episode
A depressive episode is characterised by a period of almost daily depressed mood or diminished interest in activities lasting at least two weeks accompanied by other symptoms such as difficulty concentrating, feelings of worthlessness or excessive or inappropriate guilt, hopelessness, recurrent thoughts of death or suicide, changes in appetite or sleep, psychomotor agitation or retardation and reduced energy or fatigue. The syndrome of depression must be present for at least two weeks, no history of mania, and not attributable to organic disease or psychoactive substance. The episode may be characterised as single or recurrent, mild, moderate or severe.

Dysthymic disorder
Dysthymic disorder is characterised by a persistent depressive mood (i.e. lasting two years or more), for most of the day, for more days than not. In children and adolescents, depressed mood can manifest as pervasive irritability. The depressed mood is accompanied by additional symptoms such as markedly diminished interest or pleasure in activities, reduced concentration and attention or indecisiveness, low self-worth or excessive or inappropriate guilt, hopelessness about the future, disturbed sleep or increased sleep, diminished or increased appetite or low energy or fatigue. During the first two years of the disorder, there has never been a two-week period during which the number and duration of symptoms were sufficient to meet the diagnostic requirements for a depressive episode. There is no history of manic, mixed or hypomanic episodes.

Source: International Classification of Diseases 11th Revision, WHO Geneva, www.icd.who.int.access on 11/5/21

depressive symptoms occurs relatively early in AD and can be persistent during the course of the disease. In an attempt to clarify the natural course and prevalence of depressive symptoms in AD, one study followed patients with probable AD for up to 14 years. The prevalence of depressive symptoms remained stable at approximately 40 per cent during the first few years of follow-up but then dropped significantly.

The relationship between cognitive impairment and the phenomenology of depression in older adults has been examined to determine whether patients with greater cognitive impairment were more likely to endorse specific symptoms independent of the level of depression. Overall, cognitive impairment was associated with greater depression severity. Patients with more severe levels of cognitive impairment were more likely to report greater social withdrawal. In contrast, symptoms such as lack of initiative and depressed mood were not as affected by level of cognitive impairment and were more sensitive to depression severity. Apathy, a very common feature of dementia, was found to be distinct from depression and social withdrawal.

DSM-5 includes a category of 'depression due to a general medical condition'. This diagnosis is given when the depressed mood occurs in the context of an already diagnosed medical illness that appears to be associated with depression. However, this aetiological association may be tenuous. Medical illnesses are common in older depressed people. Moreover, depression is often an antecedent or prodromal symptom of medical comorbidities and thus may be an early sign of disease, including neurological diseases, such as dementia. Conversely, depression may in itself be a risk factor for the development of certain medical illnesses, including vascular disease. On the other hand, medical disorders

Table 7.2 DSM-5 classification and diagnosis of depressive disorders – summary

Major depressive disorder
Five of the following symptoms must be present: depressed mood, diminished interest or loss of pleasure in all or almost activities, weight loss (more than 5 per cent of bodyweight), insomnia or hypersomnia, psychomotor agitation or retardation, fatigue or loss of energy, feelings of worthlessness or inappropriate guilt, diminished ability to think or concentrate, recurrent thoughts of death or suicide or a specific plan or actual suicide attempt.

At least one of the symptoms must be either depressed mood or diminished interest or pleasure. Symptoms should be present most of the day nearly every day. The syndrome should last at least two weeks, represent a change from previous functioning, cause significant distress or functional impairment, and not be a direct effect of substance use or a medical condition.

Specifiers can be coded for *single or recurrent episode, severity* (mild, moderate, or severe); *psychosis* (mood-congruent or mood-incongruent delusions or hallucinations) and *remission* (partial or full).

Persistent depressive disorder (dysthymia)
Depressed mood for more days than not accompanied by another two symptoms, including poor appetite or overeating, insomnia or hypersomnia, low energy or fatigue, low self esteem, poor concentration or feelings of hopelessness.

A duration of at least two years is required.

Bipolar 1 disorder (most recent episode depressed)
Individuals meet criteria for major depressive disorder and have a history of at least one manic episode.

Adjustment disorder with depressed mood
Individuals who develop depressed mood, tearfulness or hopelessness within three months of the occurrence of a stressor.

The syndrome should lead to great distress or disability, and should subside within six months of the removal of the stressor.

The symptoms do not represent 'normal bereavement'.

Source: Diagnostic and Statistical Manual of Mental Disorders, Fifth Edition, American Psychiatric Association, Washington DC, 2013.

may contribute to the pathophysiology of depression, especially vascular disease, as described in the following section.

There is evidence that depressed subjects report significantly greater medical comorbidity than control subjects who are not depressed. Primarily, this difference relates to the prevalence of cardiovascular illnesses, such as hypertension and atherosclerotic heart disease, but also occurs with gastrointestinal ulcers. Hypertension is more common in patients with sub-cortical ischaemic lesions.

Other evidence supporting the relationship between vascular disease and depression in late life includes the fact that 25 per cent of older individuals who experience a myocardial infarction or who are undergoing cardiac catheterisation also have major depression. Another 25 per cent of those exhibit milder depression. Furthermore, 50 per cent of patients with coronary artery disease and comorbid major depression have had at least one prior episode of major depression. In general, the greater the overall medical burden, the greater the risk of depression.

Vascular Depression Hypothesis

Following on from the association of high levels of comorbidity, particularly vascular disease in late life depression, the vascular depression hypothesis emerged. This hypothesis is supported by a number of findings, including the fact that hyperintensities on MRI scanning appear to be associated with vascular disease. Furthermore, it is late onset depression that is associated with a greater risk of vascular disease and concomitantly with deep white matter hyperintensities. Consequently, this hypothesis has proposed a number of clinical features that may be unique to vascular depression. These include a late age of onset, less depressive ideation, less insight, greater disability for the level of depression, presence of apathy and retardation and an increased prevalence of cognitive impairment, especially frontal/executive dysfunction. Finally, these patients appear to have a worse prognosis. Nevertheless, the hypothesis is not universally accepted and some counterarguments, such as the apparent lack of increase in the prevalence of depression with age despite a rising prevalence of vascular disease, have been put forward. If it is correct, the vascular depression hypothesis suggests that more aggressive treatment and prevention of cerebrovascular disease might reduce the risk of vascular depression. Specifically, antidepressants that promote ischaemic recovery, that is, those that enhance dopamine or noradrenaline activity, might be favoured in vascular depression.

Further to the association of vascular disease in late onset depression, in 2005 Baldwin and colleagues compared neurological signs in a group of individuals with late onset depression compared to healthy controls. The late onset depression group had a higher association with mild neurological abnormalities, particularly involving sub-cortical signs. They postulated that both neurodegenerative and vascular changes may be aetiologically related to this increased association with neurologic abnormalities.

Further support for the vascular depression hypothesis comes from another association: frontostriatal dysfunction in late life depression. This type of executive dysfunction is characterised by psychomotor slowing, decreased interest in outside activities and greater than expected impairment in daily function, complicated by lack of insight. Such patients generally show a poor response to antidepressant treatment and have a poor outcome.

The relationship between depression and irreversible cognitive impairment has been addressed in Chapter 3. However, reversible cognitive impairment at a time of major depression that responds to treatment still leaves these individuals with a significant risk of developing irreversible dementia – approximately 40 per cent within the first three years of follow-up. Thus, the reversible cognitive impairment associated with depression, like delirium, may very well be a harbinger of the later development of irreversible dementia.

Suicide Risk

In most epidemiologic studies, the risk of suicide is highest in elderly men. Moreover, the ratio of attempted suicide to completed suicide is lowest in older adults. Perhaps, the most important epidemiological finding is the association of depressive syndromes with suicide in older people. The vast majority (>80 per cent) of older individuals who commit suicide have had a pre-existing major depression. These people have been seen by their family doctors prior to their suicide in a large majority of cases. Unfortunately, the depressive illness is often accompanied by comorbid medical conditions which may distract the assessing doctor. Complaints of somatic symptoms, especially pain, tend to invite treatment of a somatic nature rather than antidepressant measures which may deal with the real cause. Despite the fact that mood disorders represent the most significant independent risk factor for suicide, somatic illnesses and disability, including pain, significantly increase that risk, although their effect is probably mediated by depression in a bidirectional fashion. That is, physical illness makes depression worse, and depression makes one more likely to be sensitive to physical symptoms.

Older people are more likely to use violent means of attempting suicide compared to a younger population. Although suicidal ideation generally decreases with age, the presence of suicidal thoughts does put them at a higher risk compared to younger individuals.

Suicidal ideation must be considered an independent feature of an underlying depression which requires aggressive treatment of depression even in the face of medical comorbidity. However, measures to deal with comorbid pain and treatment of underlying medical disability are still important aspects of the treatment of such individuals.

Pathophysiology

A number of brain structures have been associated with depression in late life. Alexopoulos and colleagues have consistently shown evidence of frontostriatal dysfunction, which affects both the presentation and the clinical course of late life major depression. This, in turn, leads to increased executive dysfunction and psychomotor slowing, and may explain the increased apathy.

The amygdala has been implicated in depression as it mediates emotions. Vascular disease, such as stroke and sub-cortical ischemic changes, may affect the connections between the amygdala, the medial dorsal thalamic nucleus and the orbital frontal cortex, thus predisposing to depression. Alexopoulos has postulated that the presence of comorbid and chronic medical illnesses may be associated with increased activity of the amygdala, leading to increasing secretion of cortisol and hence depression. Increased activity of the amygdala in association with inadequate cortical modulation of emotional output may contribute to depression.

Abnormalities of the hippocampus have been associated with both depression and dementia. A number of studies have shown a decreased volume of the hippocampus associated with the first episode of major depression. This may be another factor in the association of dementia and depression.

Epidemiology

It is important to distinguish between the prevalence of depressive symptoms and a major depressive episode. Epidemiologic studies show that 10–15 per cent of older adults living in the community report some depressive symptomatology. However, only about 0.5–3 per cent of the elderly population in the community are experiencing a major depressive episode at any given time. This is equivalent to an incidence of around 0.15 per cent per year. There is some suggestion that milder forms of depression are somewhat more common in older than in younger adults. However, there is no evidence to show that the incidence or prevalence of major depression increases with advancing age.

The prevalence of late life depression is higher in medical settings than in the community. Approximately 10 per cent of older adults admitted to hospitals exhibit major depression, whereas in primary care, 6–9 per cent of older adults have major depression. In nursing homes, rates of major depression approximate 12–15 per cent, while depressive *symptoms* occur in the range of 17–35 per cent among people in long-term care. These higher prevalence rates clearly are confounded by medical and neurologic comorbidity as well as increased disability in that specific population. This is consistent with the robust finding that greater medical burden increases the risk of depression.

Treatment

Before considering specific antidepressant treatments, a careful assessment of comorbidities and drug interactions must be undertaken. Given the high prevalence of medical comorbidity and the polypharmacy associated with depressive illness in older adults, potentially treatable conditions and offending drugs must be identified and addressed.

The limited available evidence suggests that older adults have a similar antidepressant treatment response as mixed-age populations. However, the anticholinergic impact of psychotropics on older adults must be considered, and consequently it is generally considered that the serotonin reuptake inhibitor class (SSRIs) or the serotonin and noradrenergic reuptake inhibitors (SNRIs) are appropriate first choice medications for an older population. A Cochrane meta-analysis noted that there were difficulties in generalising results from clinical trials into the general population. However, overall it found the efficacy of SSRIs and tricyclic antidepressants (TCAs) to be very similar. It was noted, however, that withdrawal rates from randomised controlled trials were higher for patients taking classical TCAs than those receiving SSRIs. The available studies related to older adults are confounded by small numbers, heterogeneity of the samples and a diversity of pharmacological profiles of drugs that have often been grouped together for purposes of categorisation, but in recent decades the evidence base for the use of antidepressants in the treatment of late life depression has broadened significantly. Identifying the side effect profile is compounded by the particular importance in older adults of somatic symptoms of depression as well as the comorbid medical diseases that may mimic the side effects of specific drugs. This is an issue that has received inadequate attention considering the vulnerability to somatic symptoms and side effects of this older population.

While the dictum 'start low, go slow' certainly applies to the treatment of depression in old age, it is also clear that many elderly depressed patients require similar therapeutic doses to younger adults. As long as the antidepressant is well tolerated, one should titrate the dose according to response. Second-line drugs after SSRIs or SNRIs should include moclobemide, reboxetine, agomelatine and perhaps mianserin. Classical monoamine oxidase inhibitors such as phenelzine and tranylcypromine are effective (very effective in some cases), but the dietary restrictions required for their use, their propensity to cause postural hypotension in some older patients, their toxicity in overdose and the increasing difficulty in finding reliable sources of supply have resulted in this useful class of drugs going right out of fashion during the career of the first author of this book.

In treatment resistant cases, the trial of a TCA is warranted, with nortriptyline favoured due to its better tolerability and greater evidence base for efficacy than other TCAs. There are data to support adjunctive use of lithium and/or atypical antipsychotics, such as aripiprazole, olanzapine or quetiapine, when necessary, but close monitoring for adverse effects and tolerability is required.

For milder depressions initiated by a specific stressor or those with less severity, psychotherapeutic approaches alone or combined with an antidepressant may be a reasonable first step. Available evidence suggests that cognitive behaviour therapy, supportive psychotherapy, problem-solving therapy, interpersonal psychotherapies and even psychodynamic therapy, all have some efficacy in late life depression.

Reasons why there appears to be an 'efficacy–effectiveness gap' in the older population have been reviewed (see Mulsant et al., 2003 in the further reading section at the end of this chapter). Efficacy refers to the rate of response and recovery observed under ideal research conditions, such as a randomised controlled trial. However, whether this response rate can be generalised to the real world is tempered by 'effectiveness', which is the rate of response and recovery that is reported in the 'real world' of clinical care. In older adults, this gap is contributed to by the frequent presence of comorbid medical conditions that may lead to polypharmacy and adverse events as well as a decrease in medication adherence. For example, cognitive impairment and comorbid alcoholism are frequent complications encountered when treating older adults with depression. Second, there is evidence to support the targeting of full remission of symptoms since those with residual symptoms after initial treatment tend to have a much higher rate of relapse. Consequently, the usual treatment measures apply to older adults. These include raising the dose if tolerated for longer periods of time, switching to a different antidepressant class or adding a second antidepressant or specific augmenting agent. One should always consider including a psychotherapeutic approach to individuals who have had an adequate pharmacological trial but still experience residual symptoms.

Another important initiative to reduce the 'efficacy–effectiveness gap' is by involving carers and family members who will benefit from psychoeducation around the need for ongoing treatment and long-term monitoring. This is described in detail in Chapter 2. Finally, the management of side effects in a physically and cognitively vulnerable population is especially important. Thus, the first-choice antidepressant should be the one least likely to produce side effects and, hence, the general recommendation of avoiding the anticholinergic TCAs as first-line treatments.

For refractory depressions in late life, one should consider electroconvulsive therapy (ECT) as an important treatment option, as well as the use of the traditional irreversible monoamine oxidase inhibitors (MAOIs), such as phenelzine or tranylcypromine (if available). Notwithstanding reservations noted earlier, they can be effective when other biological measures have failed. The main complication of ECT given to older people is transient cognitive impairment, but even quite frail people tolerate the anaesthetics given for ECT fairly well and it is the treatment of choice when depression is complicated by delusions, active suicidal behaviour, refusal to eat or drink or there is a strong history of prior depressive episodes that remitted only after treatment with ECT.

Trancranial magnetic stimulation (TMS) is emerging as a viable treatment option with few adverse effects for some older people who do not respond to more traditional treatments for depression. It may be valuable for both treatment of an acute depressive episode and maintenance therapy in those prone to relapse.

Outcome

Depression at any age tends to be a remitting relapsing disorder. As the length of the depressive episode is the largest factor contributing to poor long-term outcome, initial episodes should be treated energetically as soon as they present. There is evidence to suggest that recurrent episodes are less likely when prophylactic antidepressant therapy is maintained for a long term, but it is likely that the majority of people who experience one episode of late life depression will have another if they wait for long enough. For this reason, it is important that patients and their families are educated to recognise the early symptoms of a depressive relapse and advised to seek review at an early stage if such symptoms recur.

Summary

In the management of depression, as in other areas of geriatric psychiatry, the late Brice Pitt's dictum of 'general psychiatry only more so' applies. The clinician treating an older adult with depression must take into account medical illness, multiple medical and psychotropic drugs, cognitive and neurologic factors as well as the complex psychosocial history and milieu of the patient and their family.

BIPOLAR DISORDERS AND MANIA

Definition

Bipolar disorders are defined by the history or presence of a manic or hypomanic episode as outlined by ICD-11 in Table 7.3 and DSM-5 in Table 7.4.

Special Considerations

Bipolar disorder in late life is a relatively uncommon disorder and, from a public health perspective, carries less importance than the more prevalent depressive disorders. Despite its relative rarity, the study of bipolar disorder in late life does have heuristic value in order to understand why older patients become manic late in life compared to the more common early onset bipolar patients, and in turn compared to age-matched depression patients. Unfortunately, current knowledge is based primarily on retrospective cohort studies, case reports, small case series and only recently from epidemiological data using large health databases.

Classification

The high levels of medical and neurological comorbidity in the older bipolar population have clouded the diagnostic picture. This has been complicated by the classification of DSM-5, which includes a category of 'bipolar and related disorder due to a general medical condition'. This diagnosis implies that the disturbance is 'the direct pathophysiologic consequence of another medical condition'. Unfortunately, the high levels of comorbidity prevalent in late life make the assumption of 'direct pathophysiologic consequence' very difficult to ascertain. The assumption of an aetiological relationship is precarious in these circumstances.

An earlier classification, known as 'secondary mania', implied that systemic medical factors were responsible for this syndrome. Supporting evidence includes a close temporal relationship between medical/neurologic conditions and the manic syndrome. A negative family history is further support of this subtype. Others have suggested that mania in late life

Table 7.3 ICD-11 classification of bipolar disorders – summary

Bipolar type I disorder

Bipolar type I disorder is an episodic mood disorder defined by the occurrence of one or more manic or mixed episodes. A manic episode is an extreme mood state lasting at least one week, unless shortened by a treatment intervention, characterised by euphoria, irritability or expansiveness, and by increased activity or a subjective experience of increased energy, accompanied by other characteristic symptoms such as rapid or pressured speech, flight of ideas, increased self-esteem or grandiosity, decreased need for sleep, distractibility, impulsive or reckless behaviour and rapid changes among different mood states (i.e. mood lability). A mixed episode is characterised by either a mixture or very rapid alternation between prominent manic and depressive symptoms on most days during a period of at least two weeks. Although the diagnosis can be made based on evidence of a single manic or mixed episode, typically manic or mixed episodes alternate with depressive episodes over the course of the disorder.

Bipolar type II disorder

Bipolar type II disorder is an episodic mood disorder defined by the occurrence of one or more hypomanic episodes and at least one depressive episode. A hypomanic episode is a persistent mood state lasting for at least several days characterised by persistent elevation of mood or increased irritability as well as increased activity or a subjective experience of increased energy, accompanied by other characteristic symptoms such as increased talkativeness, rapid or racing thoughts, increased self-esteem, decreased need for sleep, distractibility and impulsive or reckless behaviour. The symptoms represent a change from the individual's typical mood, energy level and behaviour but are not severe enough to cause marked impairment in functioning. A depressive episode is characterised by a period of almost daily depressed mood or diminished interest in activities occurring most of the day, nearly every day during a period lasting at least two weeks, accompanied by other symptoms such as changes in appetite or sleep, psychomotor agitation or retardation, fatigue, feelings of worthless or excessive or inappropriate guilt, feelings or hopelessness, difficulty concentrating and suicidality. There is no history of manic or mixed episodes.

Source: International Classification of Diseases 11th Revision, WHO Geneva, www.icd.who.int.access on 11/5/21

resembles the neurologically defined 'disinhibition syndrome'. Affective vulnerability, be it acquired or genetic, may have been expressed in earlier life as a temperamental vulnerability. However, cerebral organic factors may unmask this vulnerability and produce a 'manic syndrome'.

Epidemiology

It is important to distinguish between the prevalence of bipolar disorder based on hospital admission rates compared to community-based surveys. For inpatient psychogeriatric units, a relatively high 'treated prevalence' of 48 per cent has been reported. Furthermore, first admission rates for mania show a modest increase at

Table 7.4 DSM-5 classification of bipolar disorders – summary

Manic episode

A. A distinct period of abnormally and persistently elevated, expansive or irritable mood, lasting at least one week (or any duration if hospitalisation is necessary).

B. During the period of mood disturbance, three or more of the following symptoms have persisted (four if the mood is only irritable) and have been present to a significant degree.

    (1) Inflated self-esteem or grandiosity

    (2) Decreased need for sleep (e.g. feels rested after only three hours of sleep)

    (3) More talkative than usual or pressure to keep talking

    (4) Flight of ideas or subjective experience that thoughts are racing

    (5) Distractibility (i.e. attention too easily drawn to unimportant or irrelevant external stimuli)

    (6) Increase in goal-directed activity (either socially, at work or school, or sexually) or psychomotor agitation

    (7) Excessive involvement in pleasurable activities that have a high potential for painful consequences (e.g. engaging in unrestrained buying sprees, sexual indiscretions or foolish business investments)

C. The mood disturbance is sufficiently severe to cause marked impairment in occupational functioning or in usual social activities or relationships with others, or to necessitate hospitalisation to prevent harm to self or others, or there are psychotic features.

D. The symptoms are not due to the effects of a substance or a medical condition.

Hypomanic episode

The episode is not severe enough to cause marked impairment in social or occupational functioning, or to necessitate hospitalisation, and there are no psychotic features.

Criteria for bipolar disorder differentiate between Bipolar 1 and 2 (the latter requiring previous lifetime diagnoses of both major depression and mania) and specify specific diagnostic rules for mild, moderate and severe degrees of illness as well as for episodes with and without psychosis and or in partial or full remission.

Source: Diagnostic and Statistical Manual of Mental Disorders, Fifth Edition, American Psychiatric Association, Washington DC, 2013.

the extremes of late life. Indeed, specialised psychogeriatric units report approximately 7–10 admissions per year. This relatively high prevalence of manic and bipolar disorders sits in stark contrast to community studies, such as the Epidemiologic Catchment Area (ECA) study, which showed a negligible prevalence of mania in people over 60 years of age who were living in the community (<0.1 per cent). This is dramatically lower than the relatively high prevalence of 1.4 per cent found in young adults. This discrepancy in community prevalence raises the question of 'where have all the young bipolars gone?' A number of theories have been posited, including the relatively high mortality rate from natural causes, an increased rate of suicide and a suggestion that in the longer term, bipolarity 'burns out'. These questions remain unanswered and may only be addressed through carefully designed prospective studies of long duration.

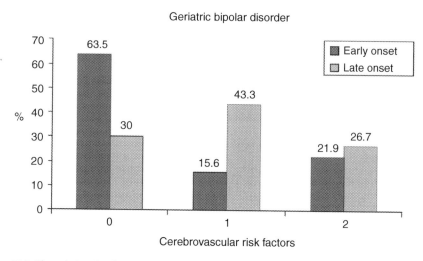

Figure 7.1 The relationship between cerebrovascular disorders and the risk of mania

Age of Onset

Age of onset remains an important variable in distinguishing subtypes of bipolarity, which in turn may reflect a different pathogenesis and aetiology. For older bipolar patients, the median age of onset tends to be around the age of 50, and this is the most commonly used cut-off point for 'late onset' disorder.

In Finland, almost 20 per cent of first admissions for bipolar disorder occur after the age of 60. In contrast, community-based samples, such as the ECA study and the US National Comorbidity Study (see Further Reading section), report mean age of onset for bipolar disorder to be the early 20s.

Using the age of 50 as the cut-off for a late onset group of bipolar patients, a significant increase in cerebrovascular risk factors was found by Wylie *et al.* (see 1999 article in the Further Reading section) (see Figure 7.1). This is not dissimilar to findings in older depressed patients where vascular depression and other vascular risk factors are significant contributing factors and comorbid phenomena. Even with late onset subjects who have a lesser family history of psychiatric disorders compared to early onset cases, the prevalence of positive family history in first-degree relatives of older bipolar patients remains higher than the general population. Moreover, aged bipolar patients have greater genetic loading than control groups with major depression only.

Neurological Comorbidity and Pathophysiology

The high prevalence of comorbid neurological disease in older bipolar patients has been a robust finding over many studies in different populations. The neurologic comorbidity has led to use of the terms 'disinhibition syndrome' and 'secondary mania'. Moreover, pathological laughing and crying, which may or may not be related to mood disorders, such as depression and mania, tend to differentiate by lesion location. Pathological laughing is associated with right-sided lesions, while left-sided lesions tend to produce pathologic crying.

The underlying pathophysiology for bipolarity may relate to the integrity of the frontal, limbic and basal ganglia circuitry, known functionally as the orbitofrontal circuit. This integrates sensory input with motivational states. Evidence primarily from the neuroimaging literature supports the hypothesis that right-sided orbitofrontal lesions mediate manic syndromes. Furthermore, a preponderance of basal temporal lesions was found in the first year following head injury (see the Jorge *et al.*, 1993 article in the Further Reading section). Patients with frontotemporal dementia, distinct from AD, present with disinhibition phenomena that may mimic mania. This is an important differential diagnostic issue but may be also relevant to understanding the underlying pathophysiology for more typical bipolar disorders. For example, in cases of dementia with disinhibition, there was a greater decrease in metabolic activity in the orbitofrontal circuit than in parietal areas. It may be that secondary mania results from disinhibition produced by lesions that disrupt connections within the orbitofrontal circuit. Frontal lobes modulate motivational and psychomotor behaviour, while limbic connections modulate emotions. Furthermore, the biogenic amine nuclei located in the amygdala, brainstem and hypothalamus may in turn modulate instinctive behaviours that are connected to the syndrome of mania.

More support for lesion location comes from a review of focal unilateral cortical lesions (see the article by Braun *et al.*, 1999 in the Further Reading section). Right-sided lesions tend to produce mania and 'pseudomania', whereas left hemisphere lesions tend to be associated with depression and 'pseudodepression'.

The extent of neurological comorbidity has been approximated in retrospective studies of late life bipolarity. Neurological comorbidity was 36 per cent in manic patients compared to only 8 per cent in age- and sex-matched patients with depression. Within the manic subgroup, a first affective episode of mania late in life was more likely to be associated with a neurological lesion (71 per cent) compared to those elderly patients who experienced multiple episodes by the time they had reached old age.

The most common neurological disorder described in the literature is cerebrovascular disease. Similar to the vascular depression hypothesis, a vascular subtype of mania has been proposed. This subtype is based on clinical and neuroimaging findings of cerebrovascular disease. Supporting clinical evidence includes a history of stroke, transient ischaemic attack (TIA) or focal signs, while positive neuroimaging includes the presence of hyperintensities or silent cerebral infarctions. Certainly, cognitive dysfunction is more common in this subgroup.

Neuroimaging

Sub-cortical hyperintensities predominate in studies of bipolar disorder, especially in late life. These sub-cortical hyperintensities reflect cerebrovascular disease. This includes hypertension, arteriosclerotic heart disease and diabetes mellitus. Late onset mania is also associated with a higher than expected prevalence of silent cerebral infarctions as found on neuroimaging. These patients tend to have a lower incidence of family history in first-degree relatives, supporting the 'vascular mania' hypothesis.

Clinical Course and Outcome

Older bipolar patients experience the onset of a mood disorder at a mean age of 50 years. Half the index patients first hospitalised for depression demonstrate a strikingly long latency (mean 15 years) prior to the onset of their first manic episode and switch to a bipolar diagnosis. Of this subgroup, approximately one-quarter have a latency of at least 25 years until first mania. This 'conversion' to a bipolar diagnosis after many years of unipolar depression is suggestive of the role that cerebral organic factors and comorbid neurologic disorders play in late life bipolar disorder.

Even though a diagnosis of bipolar disorder hinges on the presence of a single episode of mania, the vast majority of elderly bipolar patients experience a clinical course with both depressive and manic episodes. Only a small subgroup (12 per cent) meets strict criteria for a course of unipolar mania. This subgroup has an age of onset that is significantly lower compared to the larger group of older manic patients. Indeed, the unipolar manic patients are among the very few aged affective disorder patients whose illness tended to begin early in life, suggesting a unique pathogenesis.

Outcome of bipolar disorder in late life carries a significant morbidity and mortality. In one study, half of the hospitalised older manic patients had died after a mean six years of follow-up compared to only 20 per cent of aged depressed patients. Furthermore, others have found manic patients to suffer from greater morbidity, including cognitive dysfunction and cerebrovascular disease, and to have a poor prognosis.

The Determinants of Bipolar Disorder in Later Life

1. Notwithstanding a general pattern that suggests a lower genetic loading in later onset disorders of all types, the bipolar subgroup in late life still carries a significant familial prevalence of mood disorder (50–85 per cent) in first-degree relatives. However, the issue of familial affective vulnerability may be based not only on genetic factors but also on the psychological events of early life. Given the ubiquitous presence of losses in late life, it may very well be that the more important losses related to bipolarity in late life are those that occur early in an individual's development.

2. The conversion of a latent bipolar disorder after many years suggests the contribution of degenerative changes associated with normal ageing. However, the neuroimaging literature in retrospective studies points to heterogeneous brain lesions with a predominance of cerebrovascular disease associated with mania late in life. Other conditions implicated include a variety of brain tumours, alcoholism and a wide range of metabolic conditions.

3. Finally, the vulnerability to mood disorder and the presence of brain changes may not be sufficient to produce a relatively uncommon syndrome such as mania in late life. The localisation of those lesions to the right hemisphere and specifically to the orbitofrontal circuit may be the critical factor in the manifestation of this condition. Thus, localisation of brain pathology to the right-sided orbitofrontal circuit, in combination with a vulnerability to mood disorder, may constitute the pathogenetic combination necessary for the development of mania in late life.

Treatment

There have been few randomised controlled trials of pharmacological treatment in older bipolar patient populations. Consequently, clinicians often rely on guidelines designed for mixed-age populations and extrapolate from the evidence available on pharmacokinetic and pharmacodynamic changes in older adults. Atypical antipsychotics generally are used for the acute severe manic episode although efficacy studies show value for atypicals in the continuation phase too. Mood stabilisers may be introduced in the acute phase and are continued for longer periods of prophylaxis.

Lithium carbonate remains the mainstay of pharmacological treatment for bipolar disorder at all ages. However, there are special considerations regarding the use of lithium in old age, primarily related to the fact that lithium is eliminated exclusively by the kidneys, and age-associated decreases in creatinine clearance, and hence lithium clearance, affect serum lithium levels. Furthermore, pharmacodynamic factors cause an increased vulnerability to adverse reactions in an older population. Specifically, the use of drugs such as diuretics, angiotensin-converting enzyme (ACE inhibitors) and nonsteroidal anti-inflammatory drugs (NSAIDs) has been implicated in cases of lithium toxicity and increased serum levels of lithium. This is a significant concern because these drugs are so commonly prescribed to older adults. Notwithstanding the appropriate cautions associated with the use of lithium carbonate in older adults, it has remained a standard treatment for a large cohort of bipolar patients. Sudden discontinuation of lithium carbonate, especially in old age, is very likely to result in a relapse of the bipolar condition.

Pharmacoepidemiological data show a dramatic decrease in prescription patterns for lithium compared to sodium valproate/divalproex in older adults with new onset bipolar disorder. It would appear that marketing factors combined with concerns about the potential toxicity of lithium carbonate have favoured this shift in practice. Unfortunately, there is little evidence to support this trend in terms of effectiveness or safety data. For example, a population-based cohort study on the incidence of delirium in older adults found no significant difference between those treated for the first time with lithium and those treated with sodium valproate. However, treatment with lithium carbonate in older adults is associated with an increase in the development of hypothyroidism requiring thyroxine replacement (approximately 6 per cent per annum).

Despite the potential difficulties and adverse events associated with lithium carbonate in older adults, the dramatic change in prescription patterns should be reconsidered in light of its long-standing use as a mainstay treatment for bipolar disorder. In the meantime, careful monitoring of older patients on lithium is essential. Unfortunately, guidelines for serum levels are problematic in that we have little scientific basis by which to monitor serum levels, although it is clear that the therapeutic range once recommended for the younger adult population (0.5–1.2 mMol/l) is inappropriate for an older population. Clinical consensus suggests that the maintenance serum lithium level should be closer to 0.5–0.6 mMol/l, with a maximum in the 0.8 mMol/l range, above which serious side effects become very likely. Evidence suggests that long-term effective prophylaxis is unlikely with levels below 0.4 mMol/L.

Other mood stabilising agents, such as carbamazepine, lamotrigine and oxcarbazepine, have shown promising results in mixed-age bipolar patients but have not been studied in a systematic manner in older adults. Similarly, a number of atypical antipsychotic agents, such as olanzapine, risperidone and quetiapine, have shown efficacy in a mixed-age bipolar population, especially for the treatment of mania and in continuation therapy. However, there are scant data on older populations.

As highlighted in Chapter 2, the involvement of carers and family members in the management of bipolar disorder in older adults is especially important. Like all major psychiatric disorders, the family is profoundly affected by bipolar disorder and deserves attention in the management of these illnesses. Carers can guide treatment, and in turn psychoeducation for family members may improve adherence.

Summary

Bipolar disorder in older adults, as defined by an episode of mania or hypomania, represents a prototypic neuropsychiatric syndrome, which in turn reflects its neurologic basis. Nonetheless, affective vulnerability (usually genetic, sometimes psychological) is associated with the late manifestation of mania, often precipitated by heterogeneous neurologic disorders. Cerebrovascular pathology is particularly common, as evidenced clinically as well as on neuroimaging by lacunar infarcts, cortical and sub-cortical hyperintensities. The localisation of these brain lesions to the right side of the brain affecting the orbitofrontal circuit appears to be specific to late onset mania. Treatment of bipolar disorders in old age must take into account the significant comorbidity and special considerations, including decreased renal function associated with long-term lithium therapy, which has been the mainstay of bipolar treatment of the past generation. Newer pharmacological agents, including the atypical antipsychotics and anticonvulsant drugs, offer a variety of alternatives that require more formal evaluation in an older population. Involvement of family remains an essential component of ongoing management.

Further Reading

Articles

Alexopoulos, G. S. (2005). Depression in the elderly. *Lancet*, 365, 1961–1970. doi: 10.1016/S0140-6736(05)66665-2.

A clear overview from one of the most highly respected researchers in the field.

Almeida, O. (2008). Vascular depression: myth or reality? *International Psychogeriatrics*, 20, 645–652. doi: 10.1017/S1041610207006473.

An impassioned refutation of the vascular depression hypothesis.

Baldwin, R. C. and O'Brien, J. (2002). Vascular basis of late-onset depressive disorder. *British Journal of Psychiatry*, 180, 157–160. doi: 10.1192/bjp.180.2.157.

An evidence-based argument in favour of the vascular depression hypothesis.

Baldwin, R. *et al.* (2005). Neurological findings in late-onset depressive disorder: comparison of individuals with and without depression. *British Journal of Psychiatry*, 186, 308–313. doi: 10.1192/bjp.186.4.308.

An important paper suggesting a difference in the prevalence of neurologic disorders between depressed and non-depressed elderly people.

Braun, C. M. J. *et al.* (1999). Mania, pseudomania, depression, and pseudodepression resulting from focal unilateral cortical lesions. *Neuropsychiatry, Neuropsychology and Behavioral Neurology*, 12, 35–51.

Evidence to suggest that brain injury is an important predeterminant of some late life affective syndromes.

Kessler R. C. *et al.* (1997). The epidemiology of DSM-IIIR bipolar I disorder in a general population survey. *Psychological Medicine*, 27, 1079–1089. doi: 10.1017/s0033291797005333.

Data from the ECA study.

Krauthammer, C. and Klerman, G. L. (1978). Secondary mania: manic syndromes associated with antecedent physical illness or drugs. *Archives of General Psychiatry*, 35, 1333–1339.

Evidence for the association of manic syndromes with prior illness or drug use.

Mottram, P., Wilson, K. and Strobl, J. (2006). Antidepressants for depressed elderly (Review). In The Cochrane Library, Issue 1. *The Cochrane Collaboration*. Chichester: John Wiley and Sons, pp. 1–52. www.thecochranelibrary.com.

Mulsant, B. H. *et al.* (2003). Achieving long-term optimal outcomes in geriatric depression and anxiety. *CNS Spectrum*, 8, 27–34. doi: 10.1017/s1092852900008257.

Addresses the important issue of prophylaxis.

Shulman, K. I. *et al.* (1992). Mania compared with unipolar depression in old age. *American Journal of Psychiatry*, 142, 341–345. doi: 10.1176/ajp.149.3.341.

A useful comparative paper.

Shulman K. I. *et al.* (2003). Changing prescription patterns for lithium and divalproex in old age: shifting practice without evidence. *BMJ*, 326, 960–961. doi: 10.1136/bmj.326.7396.960.

An evidence-based argument in favour of the continued use of lithium for prophylaxis in bipolar disorders.

Wylie, M. E. *et al.* (1999). Age at onset in geriatric bipolar disorder. *American Journal of Geriatric Psychiatry*, 7, 77–83.

As noted above, this paper examines the issue of age of onset.

Book chapters

Mussen, L and Vasudev, A. (2020). Manic syndromes in old age. In T. Dening, A. Thomas, R. Stewart and J.-P. Taylor (eds.). *The Oxford Textbook of Old Age Psychiatry 3rd Edition*, Oxford: Oxford University Press, pp 637–654.

This chapter offers a detailed overview of mania and related issues.

Thomas, A. (2020). Depression in older people. In T. Dening, A. Thomas, R. Stewart and J.-P. Taylor (eds.). *The Oxford Textbook of Old Age Psychiatry 3rd Edition*, Oxford: Oxford University Press, pp. 595–622.

A very good summary of the existing literature.

Weissman, M. M. *et al.* (1991). Affective disorders. In L. N. Robins and D. A. Regier, *Psychiatric Disorders in America: the Epidemiologic Catchment Area Study*, New York: Free Press, pp. 53–90.

Good, if dated overview of the relevant epidemiology from the largest such study ever conducted.

Book

Moulds, R. *et al.* (2013). *Therapeutic Guidelines: Psychotropic, Version 7*. Melbourne: Therapeutic Guidelines.

This very useful text contains excellent sections on the evidence-based treatment of both depression and mania, with some consideration of issues affecting older patients. The table giving details for crossover times when changing antidepressants is very helpful in clinical practice. It is likely that a new edition will be published before the end of 2022.

Schizophrenia and Related Disorders in Late Life

Brief Historical Notes

Most health professionals have some familiarity with the diagnosis of schizophrenia and psychoses occurring in young adults. For people with psychosis in late life, the term 'late paraphrenia' had some currency from the 1950s until around 10 years ago.

Kraepelin, in his introduction to his classic text *Dementia Praecox and Paraphrenia* (English translation 1919), distinguished between dementia praecox and paraphrenia, which he described thus:

> [T]hose forms have been singled out and placed together subsequently which are distinguished in their whole course by very definite manifestations of peculiar disturbances of intellect while lacking enfeeblement of volition and especially of feeling, or at least such symptoms are only feebly indicated. It seems to be that the term 'paraphrenia', which is now no longer in common use, is in the meantime suitable as the name of morbid forms thus delimited which are here by way of experiment brought together.

Manfred Bleuler studied 126 patients whose psychosis began after 40 years of age. He noted that of these 126, 4 per cent had onset after they were 60 years old. He reported that about 50 per cent of these had symptoms which were no different from those patients whose illness began at a younger age.

In the United Kingdom, the term 'late paraphrenia' was introduced in the 1950s by Roth to describe some schizophrenia-like conditions first appearing in those over the age of 60. This term was current up to the International Classification Diseases, Version 9 (ICD-9) (1980), but was not included in ICD-10 or ICD-11.

Since the 1960s, there has been much discussion and debate regarding the nature and classification of late onset psychosis, the central issues being the following:

(a) Is this the same as schizophrenia in younger adults, but occurring later in old age?

(b) Is this biologically similar or different to schizophrenia in the younger adults?

(c) Is late onset psychosis a result of the interaction between schizophrenia and the multiple vulnerability factors associated with old age?

(d) Is late paraphrenia the end product of an ongoing psychosis?

To address these issues and resolve the controversy, an international consensus meeting was held at Leeds Castle, Kent, United Kingdom, in July 1998; this was updated in 2000. The following consensus statement was agreed upon by the expert participants after review of the literature and research to date:

'(a)Late onset schizophrenia (LOS) (illness onset after 40 years of age but otherwise indistinguishable from schizophrenia starting at an earlier age) and,

(b) Very-late-onset schizophrenia-like psychosis (VLOSP) (onset after 60 years). This latter group is generally associated with a somewhat different symptom profile and does not seem to have genetic risk factors for schizophrenia.'

They also reported that schizophrenia-like psychosis, which is not attributed to either an affective disorder or brain abnormality, can occur anytime in the life cycle, with symptoms being the most heterogeneous at the extremes of age.

Early Onset Schizophrenia: The Evolution of This Disorder with Advancing Age

Kraepelin conceptualised inevitable and inexorable deterioration in personality and psychosocial functioning as being a core part of dementia praecox (later renamed as schizophrenia by Bleuler). However, long-term studies have identified that although schizophrenia can be chronic, disabling and with outcome worse than other mental disorders, improvement and/or recovery can occur in half to two-thirds of cases. The movement towards de-institutionalisation (complete in many high-income countries) and the continued ageing of the 'baby boomer' cohort will result in more 'graduates' (people with life-long schizophrenia who have grown old) living in the community requiring treatment, support and management from specialist old age psychiatry services.

The ongoing psychotic symptoms of chronic schizophrenia in late life age are usually a continuation of what has appeared in the patient's earlier years – delusions, hallucinations (usually auditory) and thought disorder. These may be attenuated in intensity and frequency by time and treatment. The ageing process itself, in entering developmental maturity, may exert an ameliorating effect on the symptoms.

However, ongoing negative symptoms of avolition, blunted affect, deterioration of personality and psychosocial function, such as described by Kraepelin, may, when present, become more severe. The confounding effects of depression, psychosocial isolation resulting from many years of negative symptomatology combined with demoralisation, lack of social support, long periods of hospitalisation and continuous use of antipsychotic medication negatively impact on their quality of life and thus make negative symptoms appear to be more severe and disabling.

The emergence of cognitive impairment in old age will further compound these problems, thus creating a 'double jeopardy'. Although some old people with schizophrenia may be entering a dementing process, it is to be noted that not all cognitive impairment in these patients represents dementia and may be due to incident delirium, the cognitive symptoms of schizophrenia itself or other causes, such as medication use or depression.

Schizophrenia with Onset in Late Life

As many studies in late life schizophrenia were done prior to the Leeds Castle consensus meeting, and only a few have been published since 1998, our knowledge of the condition, which that meeting defined as VLOSP, is emerging only slowly.

Clinical Features

Phenomenologically, delusions and hallucinations can emerge for the first time at any age; other features of schizophrenia, such as thought disorder, affective blunting and avolition, appear to become less frequent with increasing age. 'Partition delusions' (relating to the phantom presence of hallucinatory voices or noises emanating from the floors, ceilings or

Table 8.1 Clinical presentation of schizophrenia in late life

Early onset	Late onset
Delusions	Delusions
• Systematised	• Systematised
• Non-systematised	• 'Partition'
	• Phantom boarders
Hallucinations	Hallucinations
• Usually auditory	• Multi-modal
Thought disorder	Thought disorder
• Common	• Uncommon
Negative symptoms	Negative symptoms
• Common	• Uncommon

(from Hassett *et al.* 2005).

walls of one's abode) with persecutory themes are more prominent in old age. Table 8.1 summarises the contrasting presentations.

Epidemiology

While there are multiple methodological issues in studies reporting epidemiological data in late onset schizophrenia, a general picture can be obtained.

The Ageing and Liverpool Health Aspects Study with a sample of 5,222 community subjects reported a prevalence of 0.12 per cent. The Epidemiological Catchment Area (ECA) study in the United States reported a one-year prevalence rate of 0.6 per cent in subjects between 45 and 64 years and 0.2 per cent for those over 65 years.

There is a strong predominance of females in late onset schizophrenia ranging from a high 22.5:1 female:male ratio to a low 1.6:1 ratio, suggesting a particular vulnerability in women for first onset of a psychotic illness in late life.

Risk factors, apart from the obvious genetic factors, include the contribution of sensory impairment, social isolation and premorbid personality with prominent paranoid/schizoid traits.

Neuroimaging in Late Onset Schizophrenia

To try to understand the pathological processes in the development of LOS and VLOSP, neuroimaging is potentially a useful tool in studies of this condition. However, at this stage of neuroimaging technology and research, the findings in LOS are similar to that of EOS, which include increased Ventricular Brain Ratio (VBR) and reduction in Regional Blood Flow (RBF) in the temporal area. The role of white matter hyperintensities (WMHs) is unclear, and the increasing amounts seen in LOS could also be due to the natural accumulation of these seen in older age. Functional imaging has found hypoperfusion in various areas, such as the frontal and temporal regions, but these findings have not been consistent. PET and SPECT studies have been inconclusive with both increased and no increase in D2 receptors, compared to controls. The technologies of fMRI, MRS and MEG may in the future help elucidate possible aetiologies in late onset schizophrenia.

Cognitive Change in Late Onset Schizophrenia

Cognitive impairment is part of the clinical characteristics of schizophrenia, both in EOS and LOS and is generally similar. The cognitive impairment is static and occasionally reversible with treatment. This contrasts with that of neurodegenerative disorders such as dementia – late onset patients will have preserved learning capacity, which is in contrast to those with Alzheimer's disease (AD).

Neuropsychological studies have demonstrated that LOS is not associated with senile plaques or obvious amyloid pathology, suggesting that the neuropathological processes of LOS and AD are distinct.

Studies to date have not found a disproportionately higher rate of cognitive decline or dementia amongst LOS subjects.

Management of Late Onset Schizophrenia and 'Graduates' with Long-standing Early Onset Schizophrenia

Physical Management

As medical comorbidity is the rule rather than the exception in late life, the identification and energetic treatment of such conditions is a priority. The management of general physical health will benefit all patients with schizophrenia. The collaboration of a family physician and/or specialist geriatricians/physicians will enhance this aspect of management.

'Graduates' who have been disabled by schizophrenia for many years may have neglected their physical health and may not have had consistent health maintenance. Therefore, close attention should be given to this aspect in assessment and any outstanding issues should be actively pursued.

For those who develop schizophrenia in late life, and who have had good health maintenance up to date, this should be encouraged to be continued. Sensory impairment should be addressed if possible.

Pharmacological Management

For 'graduates' who are continuing their pharmacological management, consistent and constant monitoring of compliance, adverse effects and the interaction with other drugs should be a high priority. Any change of medication will need to take into consideration the alteration in physiological status of an older person and the effects on development of adverse events. At least one study has shown that patients on classical antipsychotics whose symptoms are not well controlled or who experience significant side effects from these medications may benefit when their treatment is switched to olanzapine or risperidone.

To start treatment for LOS, and particularly VLOSP, atypical antipsychotics (olanzapine, risperidone, quetiapine, aripiprazole etc.) are the drugs of choice. Efficacy of these medications has been adequately demonstrated in trials including younger patients, but there is a paucity of data to guide the prescriber whose patients are elderly. They do reduce core symptoms of schizophrenia, have low extrapyramidal side effects and are much better tolerated than conventional (typical) antipsychotics. The choice between available atypical antipsychotics is not at all clear and there is little evidence to support the use of one over the other in relation to efficacy or the emergence of such adverse effects as motor disorders, although each has marginal and different adverse events in other domains. Doses prescribed should be as low as possible (e.g. 1–4 mg risperidone daily, 2.5–15 mg olanzapine daily), while achieving a therapeutic effect. In practice, the optimum dose to be used will need to be determined for each patient, with factors such as symptom control and the presence of dose-dependent adverse effects being pre-eminent. Some patients will do poorly on one drug and better on another. Not every patient will respond to treatment; studies of classical anti-psychotics suggest that one-quarter to one-third of patients with LOS and VLOSP receive no net benefit from antipsychotic therapy and only one-quarter achieve complete remission. Nevertheless, even a modest amelioration of symptoms may allow a supervised return to independent living in the community.

Some studies have suggested that older patients may be at higher risk of adverse effects such as tardive dyskinesia and extrapyramidal side effects, so these need to be carefully monitored for.

Psychosocial Management

The psychosocial needs of this group of patients who are increasingly living independently in the community highlight the necessity to develop multidisciplinary comprehensive management strategies to improve their quality of life in conjunction with effective symptom reduction through energetic pharmacological treatment.

As they have multiple, complex needs, resulting from a combination of physical psychological and psychotic symptoms in late life, the strategies of case management combined with individual service plans in consultation with the patient and any significant family members should underpin their care. This will provide holistic and comprehensive support, taking care of all the psychosocial and physical aspects of their lives.

Residential Care

As these patients age and their functional capacity declines, consideration for residential care would require careful consultation to achieve the best quality of life at this later stage of their lives.

As most residential care services for the older person are planned for frail old people and those with dementia as the major consumer groups, aged patients with schizophrenia may not be appropriately located in such facilities. Special consideration will need to be made for this group of patients requiring residential care, and preferably, discussion with the unit manager, treating clinician and family should occur. Discussion about past history, symptoms, early warning signs and possible education for the facility staff may assist with transition. The development of specialist psychogeriatric nursing homes, such as exist in Victoria, Australia, to cater for this group of patients, may be a model to consider.

Other Conditions Which May Exhibit Psychotic Symptoms (Also See Chapters 5, 6, 7 and 10)

Psychotic symptoms occurring for the first time in late life frequently pose a diagnostic and management dilemma for the clinician. Table 8.2 illustrates a comparison of psychotic symptoms across life stages.

Psychotic symptoms occur frequently in elderly people with delirium. As indicated in Chapter 6, this tends to be under-recognised and was not given adequate weight in DSM-IV,

Table 8.2 Psychotic symptoms across life stages

	Young	Middle age	Old age
Schizophrenia	+	+	+
Affective disorders	+	+	++
Alcohol misuse	+	++	+
Illicit substance use	++	+	
Delusional disorder		+	+
Specific organic		+	++
Delirium			++
Dementia			++

(from Hassett *et al.* 2005).

which did not include delusions as one of the features of delirium. Many older adults who are hospitalised for medical conditions are at risk of delirium and it is important that they are adequately assessed in a timely manner with appropriate treatment. Because anti-psychotics may be prescribed during this period, follow-up with the GP is essential after discharge to review the ongoing need for the antipsychotic.

Older people with depressive illnesses also can present with psychotic symptoms, which may be mood congruent with the content of delusions and hallucinations being consistent with the depressive themes of guilt, personal deprecation, nihilism or deserved punishment for exaggerated past sins (see Chapter 7). Electroconvulsive therapy is often indicated in psychotic depression and is an efficacious treatment in the older population when judiciously used. Mania, whether it is part of an ongoing primary bipolar disorder or secondary to pathology related to central nervous system disorders, can include psychotic features of grandiose delusions, inappropriate sexual expression and paranoid response if prevented from acting out behaviours resulting from these psychotic symptoms.

Psychotic features in dementia are well recognised and have been extensively researched (see Chapter 5). In older persons presenting with psychotic symptoms for the first time, dementia should always be kept in mind and vigorously explored.

The presence of psychotic symptoms in specific neurological disorders, such as basal ganglia disorders (especially Parkinson's disease) and cerebrovascular disease, should be noted. Adverse psychotic reactions to drugs used to treat Parkinson's disease occur quite frequently.

Iatrogenic Substance-Induced Causes of Psychotic Symptoms

One of the very common causes of psychotic symptoms in the elderly is the adverse effect of both prescribed and over-the-counter preparations. Anticholinergic drugs, dopamine agonists, opiates, corticosteroids, tricyclic antidepressants, low potency conventional antipsychotics, non-steroidal inflammatory drugs and digoxin are well known high-risk drugs for the causation of delirium and psychotic features in late life. Benzodiazepines, beta-blocking drugs and calcium channel-blocking agents have lower but nevertheless significant risks attached to their use.

Medication monitoring and constant review by clinicians is an essential best practice in the management of all older patients.

Conclusion

While the concept and classification of schizophrenia are still under continuing review, the distress of psychotic symptoms to older people and their families should cause all clinicians to take the greatest care in the identification and management of these symptoms, whether they be due to schizophrenic spectrum disorders or to other possible causes.

Further Reading

Articles

Howard, R. *et al.* (2000). Late onset schizophrenia – very late onset schizophrenia-like psychosis: an international consensus. *American Journal of Psychiatry*, 157, 172–178. doi: 10.1176/appi.ajp.157.2.172.

The current international consensus on classifying this complex group of disorders.

Jeste, D. V. *et al.* (1999). Conventional versus newer antipsychotics in the elderly. *American Journal of Geriatric Psychiatry*, 7, 70–76.

A balanced view of the pharmacological treatment options.

Ritchie, C. *et al.* (2003). The impact upon extra-pyramidal side effects, clinical symptoms and quality of life of a switch from conventional to atypical antipsychotics (Risperidone or Olanzapine) in elderly patients with schizophrenia. *International Journal of Geriatric Psychiatry*, 18, 432–440. doi: 10.1002/gps.862.

Ritchie, C. *et al.* (2006). A comparison of the efficacy and safety of olanzapine and risperidone in the treatment of elderly patients with schizophrenia: an open study of six months duration. *International Journal of*

Geriatric Psychiatry, 21, 171–179. doi: 10.1002/gps.1446.

These two papers offer supportive evidence for the safety and efficacy of switching the treatment of elderly patients with schizophrenia from conventional antipsychotics to olanzapine or risperidone.

Book

Hassett, A., Ames, D. and Chiu E. (2005). *Psychosis in the Elderly*, London: Taylor and Francis.

A detailed and comprehensive overview of all forms of psychosis affecting the elderly.

Book chapter

Lee EE, Hou B, Vahia IV and Jeste DV (2020). Late onset schizophrenia. In T. Dening, A. Thomas, R. Stewart and J.-P. Taylor (eds.). *Oxford Textbook of Old Age Psychiatry, 3nd edition*, Oxford: Oxford University Press, pp 671–694.

In all editions of this famous textbook, the chapter on late onset schizophrenia has offered a superb, historically informed overview of schizophrenia and related disorders in late life, and this new version does not disappoint.

Chapter

9

Neurotic and Personality Disorders

NEUROTIC DISORDERS

Introduction

Neurotic disorders are characterised by the psychological and somatic symptoms of anxiety and depression, complicated by various maladaptive attempts to manage and control these symptoms, such as phobic avoidance and somatisation. These conditions are the most common mental disorders at all ages, and they incur substantial direct and indirect costs to health and social services. Despite the fact that neurotic disorders are relatively prevalent in the older population, they tend not to present to services, or are missed or misdiagnosed if they do. This is a pity, because in many cases they are significantly distressing and disabling, and they are potentially treatable.

The Concept of Neurosis

The unitary and dimensional concept of neurosis that developed over the eighteenth and nineteenth centuries has given way in the modern era to a wide range of discretely defined categorical disorders, currently enshrined in the ICD-11 and DSM-5 classifications (Table 9.1). This categorical approach to illness is congenial to the modern case-oriented way of medical thinking, involving as it does decision making, discriminating, service planning and the organising of reimbursement and research. However, it does not follow therefore that all forms of illness conform to this model, and there is good evidence that neurotic disorders are related to each other in important and fundamental ways. For example, there is extensive comorbidity between this group of disorders and between them and depression, and follow-up studies demonstrate that there is also considerable movement of individuals between diagnostic categories over time. Perhaps most importantly, diagnosis does not appear to be particularly helpful in predicting response to specific forms of treatment. What the two-dimensional categories of ICD-11 and DSM-5 fail to capture is the reality of common mental disorders as *processes*, the complex and variable outcome of interactions between individual vulnerability, circumstances and inappropriate and self-defeating responses to distress. This is particularly important for understanding older patients, who often come with a lifetime's experience of their condition and its consequences.

The Aetiology of Neurotic Disorders

According to Goldberg and Huxley (see the Further Reading section for details of their influential 1992 text), all neurotic disorders are grounded in the core experiences of anxiety

Table 9.1 Current classifications of neurotic disorders

ICD-11	DSM-5
Mood disorders	**Mood disorders**
F34: *Persistent mood disorders*	*Depressive disorders*
Dysthymia	300.4: Persistent depressive disorder (Dysthymia)
Neurotic, stress-related and somatoform disorders	
F40: *Phobic anxiety disorders*	**Anxiety disorders**
.0: Agoraphobia	300.01: Panic disorder
.1: Social phobia	300.22: Agoraphobia
.2: Specific phobia	300.23: Social anxiety disorder (social phobia)
	300.29: Specific phobia
F41: *Other anxiety disorders*	300.3: Obsessive-compulsive disorder
	309.81: Post-traumatic stress disorder
.0: Panic disorder	300.02: Generalised anxiety disorder
.1: Generalised anxiety disorder	293.84: Anxiety disorder due to another general medical condition
.2: Mixed anxiety and depressive disorder	Substance-induced anxiety disorder
F42: *Obsessive-compulsive disorder*	
F43: *Reaction to severe stress, and*	
adjustment disorders	
.0: Acute stress reaction	
.1: Post-traumatic stress disorder	
.2: Adjustment disorders	
F44: *Dissociative disorders*	**Dissociative disorders**
.0: Dissociative amnesia	300.12: Dissociative amnesia
.1: Dissociative fugue	300.13: Dissociative fugue
.2: Dissociative stupor	300.14: Dissociative identity disorder
.3: Trance and possession states	300.6: Depersonalisation disorder
.4: Dissociative motor disorders	
.5: Dissociative convulsions	
.6: Dissociative anaesthesia and sensory loss	
F45: *Somatoform disorders*	**Somatic symptom disorders**
.0: Somatisation disorder	300.82: Somatic symptom disorder

Table 9.1 (cont.)

.1: Undifferentiated somatoform disorder	300.11: Conversion disorder
.2: Hypochondriacal disorder	300.7: Illness anxiety disorder
.3: Somatoform autonomic dysfunction	300.7: Body dysmorphic disorder
.4: Persistent somatoform pain disorder	300.19 Factitious disorder
F46: *Other neurotic disorders*	
.0: Neurasthenia	
.1: Depersonalisation-derealisation syndrome	

and depression, which in turn reflect the activity of specific neuronal systems in response to reward and punishment. A number of factors determine whether and when an individual develops an episode of illness, and the subsequent course of that episode.

Vulnerability Factors

These factors determine an individual's general liability to develop psychological symptoms in response to adverse experiences. Genetic factors appear to have a diagnostically non-specific effect in increasing the risk of neurotic disorder, perhaps by determining emotional reactivity; the personality trait of 'neuroticism' is under significant genetic control. Across the lifespan, environmental and psychosocial factors such as early parental loss, limited education, chronic social adversity, limited social networks, low levels of social support and physical disability, all increase vulnerability to neurotic disorders. Some factors, such as the impact of physical illness and disability, probably have a greater impact as vulnerability factors in older age. Environmental factors experienced during childhood may determine future vulnerability through their effect on personality development, in particular the favoured cognitive defence styles in the face of threat and loss. Factors experienced in adulthood, such as long-standing social adversity, may act by increasing low self-esteem, or by increasing individuals' vulnerability to other factors, such as physical ill health and other adverse life events.

Destabilisation Factors

These factors are the experiences that provoke the onset of psychological symptoms in sufficiently vulnerable individuals. The impact of adverse life events has been extensively researched at all ages, and it has been shown that experiences involving loss and threat are important in relation to the onset of depression and anxiety, respectively. It is the meaning of the event to the individual, not its objective severity, that matters most in terms of its liability to provoke illness. Some types of life events, such as retirement, bereavement and institutionalisation, occur more frequently in old age, and might therefore be important causes of anxiety and depression in this age group, but the evidence is by no means clear on this point. The 'timeliness' of such events in late life may reduce their impact, as may the degree of planning, preparation and choice involved.

Some extreme and catastrophic experiences, such as major accidents, wars or natural disasters, have the potential to provoke significant psychological distress in all but the most robust individuals. In ICD-11 and DSM-5, the close relationship between trauma and the psychological response to it has led to these stress reactions being classified as separate diagnoses, notably post-traumatic stress disorder (PTSD); they are discussed further in the following sections.

Restitution Factors

These factors determine the duration of psychological symptoms, and the nature of the recovery from them. Sometimes the restitution from an episode of illness is uncomplicated, with individuals making a full recovery. Several factors contribute to successful restitution, including the nature of the episode (mild rather than severe), resolution of the provoking life event, crisis support, 'fresh start' events and the lack of other complicating vulnerability factors, like chronic social adversity and poor social networks. Mental health services can also contribute to the successful resolution of illness in many cases, as many of the randomised controlled trials of psychotropic drugs and psychological interventions against placebo have shown.

In some cases, the restitution from an episode of illness can be complicated by the development of damaging and disabling distress-management strategies, such as phobic avoidance, self-medication with alcohol and other drugs, re-labelling as physical illness and so on. If these persist, they can lead to the enduring clusters of symptoms and behaviour that we recognise as specific neurotic disorders (agoraphobia, somatisation disorder etc.).

Epidemiology

Comparisons between epidemiological studies are difficult, because the different rules employed with regard to symptom definition, severity and diagnostic hierarchies result in very different rates of these disorders. Some generally applicable findings from community population surveys include a fall in prevalence and incidence rates with increasing age across the adult lifespan, and a female preponderance for most disorders at all ages. Most older people with neurotic disorders developed them before their 50s, but elderly cases of phobic disorder, panic and obsessive-compulsive disorder (OCD) tend to be of later onset. Epidemiological studies have also identified a range of risk factors associated with neurotic disorders in older populations, such as female gender, ethnic group, physical illness and disability and various markers of social adversity, such as dependency on state benefits.

Clinical Features

The psychological and somatic symptoms and disturbances of behaviour associated with these disorders are broadly similar at all ages, but in older patients there may be differences in how they are expressed or perceived by others. In this age group, the clinical challenge is to be appropriately alert to the possibility of neurotic disorder, without misattributing potentially significant and serious symptoms of underlying physical illness.

Psychological Symptoms

As already mentioned, this group of disorders is characterised by an admixture of depressive and anxiety symptoms. Depressive symptomatology in late life is discussed in detail in Chapter 7. When other factors are taken into account, older people appear to worry less than younger people, but if they do, it is more likely to be associated with mental disorder; significant worry in old age should therefore not be dismissed but instead prompt further assessment of the mental state. Similarly, clinically important fears expressed by elderly people are sometimes regarded as reasonable on the grounds of age alone; in fact, it is issues such as frailty and the availability of social support that are more important in determining these individuals' perceptions of vulnerability and risk.

The clinical features and phenomenology of obsessive compulsive disorder (OCD) are also similar to those seen in younger patients. It is rare for OCD to have its onset in later life, although cases have been reported. More commonly, diagnoses of OCD made for the first time in old age are chronic disorders that have never been adequately assessed or treated (see later in the chapter).

Somatic Symptoms

The somatic symptoms of anxiety are also similar at all ages and include autonomic symptoms, muscular tension pains and headaches, motor restlessness, dyspnoea, *globus hystericus* and the physical effects of hyperventilation. In older patients however, there is much greater opportunity for misdiagnosis, medicalisation and unnecessary investigations; panic attacks are particularly prone to being referred on to cardiologists, neurologists and gastroenterologists. This probably contributes significantly to the burden of heathcare costs associated with these disorders in old age. There is also the difficulty of identifying and managing somatic anxiety symptoms in older patients with significant coexisting physical illness, such as individuals with chronic respiratory disease trapped in a vicious circle of anxiety and breathlessness. It is quite understandable why doctors should wish to investigate and refer such patients with unexplained physical symptoms; in view of the strong association between neurotic disorders and physical ill health in old age, there is always the concern that there might be an important hidden physical cause. Some suggestions to guide clinical decision making in this tricky area are given in the section Differential Diagnosis later in the chapter.

Somatisation, or the expression of psychosocial distress in the form of physical symptoms, is a common phenomenon at all ages and in all cultures, and is the commonest means by which patients with a psychiatric disorder present to primary healthcare. Despite the popular stereotype of the older patient preoccupied with their bowels or other bodily symptoms, it does not appear that somatisation is more prevalent in old age than in younger adulthood. In older psychiatric populations, it is particularly associated with anxiety and depression, and also with physical illness. It is usually managed by reassurance, and treatment of the underlying physical and psychological disorders. Most patients will understand and accept their misattribution of symptoms when this is explained, but a few do not; among these are individuals who meet criteria for a somatoform or somatisation disorder (see later in the chapter).

Hysterical symptoms are an important exception to the general observation that the clinical significance of neurotic symptoms is similar in both younger and more elderly patients. As a rule, hysterical illness does not begin in old age. Apparently, hysterical conversion reactions and dysmnesia are occasionally seen in elderly patients in response to stress, but such symptoms are usually due either to underlying undiagnosed physical illness or to the release of dissociative tendencies in vulnerable personalities by organic cerebral pathology or functional psychiatric disorder.

Patients with clinically significant anxiety commonly present with complaints of delayed or interrupted sleep due to worry and nightmares. This may be more of a problem for older patients, whose sleep architecture is subject to normal age-related changes, making sleep lighter and more prone to interruption. Individuals with sleep disturbance associated with a neurotic disorder also are prone to have difficulties with chronic hypnotic drug and alcohol use.

Behavioural Disturbance

Most of the behavioural problems associated with anxiety and depression represent maladaptive attempts to control these unpleasant experiences (q.v. Restitution factors, earlier in the chapter): phobic avoidance, substance abuse, cigarette smoking, deliberate self-harm, eating disorders and the abnormal illness behaviour associated with somatisation. In older patients with chronic neurotic disorders, these behavioural problems are likely to be of long-standing and associated with significant adverse physical and psychological consequences. In some individuals with a past history of an eating disorder or deliberate self-harm in early adulthood, the re-emergence of these problems in late life may indicate difficulty in adjusting to old age.

Differential Diagnosis

Depression

As noted, the origins of neurotic disorders and depression are closely related, and admixtures of depressive and anxiety symptoms are among the most frequent presentations, particularly in primary care settings. Therefore, the proper diagnostic question is not 'Is it depression or anxiety?', but 'How much of each?'. Indeed, in older patients, the occurrence of generalised anxiety in the absence of significant depression is the exception rather than the rule. This has important implications for management, as the primary target for intervention may be the depression rather than the anxiety (see later in the chapter).

Dementia

With the growth of memory clinics and the availability of antidementia drugs, increasing numbers of patients of all ages are referred to specialist services with complaints of impairment in their cognitive function. A key diagnostic challenge in this group is to distinguish between organic and functional causes of this impairment. 'Pseudodementia' associated with a severe depressive illness is well recognised, but subjective cognitive inefficiency can also be caused by much milder levels of both depression and anxiety, and may well be the presenting complaint in some cases. This differential diagnosis is complicated by the fact that a dementia can sometimes be heralded by episodes of anxiety and depression. In some cases, detailed neuropsychological assessment can help by finding a pattern of impairment indicative of either a functional or an organic disorder, but it is not uncommon for both this and other investigations to be uninformative. In these patients, the best course of action is to treat the functional symptoms, establish optimum baseline cognitive functioning and reassess this in a year.

A diagnosis of dementia is a major life event, and it is quite common for individuals to develop significant secondary symptoms of anxiety and depression, particularly in the early stages when insight is preserved. There is loss of confidence, worry about the future and about the family, increased irritability and social withdrawal due to fear of humiliating lapses in public. Anxiety and depression may also be more directly due to the underlying cause of the dementia, such as cerebrovascular disease (q.v.).

Delirium

Delirium is usually a quiet disorder in elderly patients, but sometimes they present with a hyperactive profile, including increased arousal, irritability and fear and aggression secondary to hallucinations and delusions. This can be mistaken for a panic attack, but an informant history and an examination of the mental state will usually reveal the underlying cause. In an older individual, such a presentation should be regarded as delirium until proved otherwise, particularly if the patient is also cognitively impaired and physically ill (see Chapter 6).

Schizophrenia

Older people with functional psychoses sometimes find their hallucinatory experiences and imagined persecutions very frightening and upsetting, but this is unlikely to cause any diagnostic difficulty (see Chapter 8). Sometimes the patient's complaints need cross-checking: is this eccentric, isolated old man deluded, or is it true that children are breaking into his flat to taunt him?

Physical Illness

Physical illness is strongly associated with anxiety and depression in old age: as a cause, as a consequence and as a mimic of these disorders. The clinical task is to delineate carefully the physical and psychological problems that are present, and the nature and extent of any relationship between them. A physical examination, ECG and routine screening laboratory investigations will pick up most of the more common primary physical causes of neurotic symptoms in elderly patients, such as myocardial infarction, cardiac arrythmia, heart failure, obstructive lung disease, endocrine and metabolic disorders, anaemia and vitamin deficiencies. If the patient is or has been a smoker, a chest X-ray is useful to rule out occult lung cancer. Symptoms of anxiety may also be secondary to prescribed medications (hypoglycaemics, corticosteroids, sympathomimetics, dopamine agonists, SSRIs), or to drug withdrawal. If this routine physical screen draws a blank, should one proceed to more detailed investigations or specialist referral? One should be more suspicious of a primary cause for neurotic symptoms in old age if they appear in individuals without any past psychiatric history, and without a clear external cause such as an adverse life event or ongoing difficulties. Neurotic symptoms with a primary physical cause usually respond to treatment of the underlying disorder, but may need managing in their own right if the illness has been severe or prolonged.

Sleep Disorders

At all ages, depression and anxiety are the commonest causes of disturbed sleep and need to be considered in any patient who presents with this problem. Other causes of sleep disturbance in older patients include insomnia due to pain and physical disability, periodic leg movements syndrome and restless legs syndrome and sleep apnoea. Sudden changes of environment, such as hospitalisation or institutionalisation, usually result in at least a transient insomnia.

Some Specific Neurotic Disorders

Generalised Anxiety Disorder (GAD)

GAD is characterised by persistent anxious mood accompanied by motor tension, autonomic symptoms, apprehensiveness and hypervigilance. Prevalence estimates of GAD in older populations range from about 1 per cent to 5 per cent. It has a chronic fluctuating course and is frequently comorbid with depression. A significant proportion of older cases appear to be of late onset, associated with functional limitations due to physical disability. GAD is also a response to severe health events, such as myocardial infarct and stroke; follow-up studies indicate that in many cases this anxiety becomes chronic, associated with poor functional outcomes.

Phobic Disorders

Phobias are defined as the persistent and irrational fear of an object, activity or situation resulting in a compelling desired to avoid the phobic stimulus. Phobic disorders are the most common anxiety disorders in late life, with one-month prevalence rates of 5–10 per cent. While many phobic disorders are long-standing, a significant proportion of agoraphobias in old age are of late onset, often in response to a traumatic event, such as an episode of physical illness, a fall, a road accident or being a victim of crime.

Panic Disorder

Panic disorder is characterised by recurrent attacks of intense fear, accompanied by severe somatic anxiety symptoms. Little is known about panic disorder in old age, but evidence from case reports, volunteer samples and non-psychiatric populations suggest that its frequency declines with age, and that late onset cases are symptomatically less severe than those whose disorder started earlier in life.

Obsessive-Compulsive Disorder (OCD)

OCD is characterised by obsessive thoughts and/or compulsive acts which are a significant source of distress, or interfere with social functioning. Although OCD is currently classified as one of the anxiety disorders, it is rather different from them in being a relatively stable diagnosis over time and having a more substantial genetic component in its aetiology. The compulsive behaviours of OCD are similar to the stereotypies seen in disorders such as Tourette's syndrome and Sydenham's chorea. OCD tends to appear in young adulthood, and it is unusual for first onset to occur after the age of 50 years. However, it is a chronic and recurrent disorder and a significant proportion of cases may present to services for the first time in old age. The late onset of obsessional symptoms may form part of a primary affective disorder, or there may be an organic cause such as dementia or a space-occupying lesion affecting the frontal lobes. The anxious orderliness associated with the onset of dementia tends not to be associated with the tension that is typical of OCD.

Post-traumatic Stress Disorder

PTSD occurs following exposure to an extreme stressor, and the syndrome includes re-experiencing of the trauma, avoidance, numbing and increased arousal. Little is known about PTSD in late life, but the disorder can persist for years, sometimes manifesting for the first time in old age.

Somatoform Disorders

Somatic symptom (somatoform) disorders in late life are poorly understood. Very few individuals of any age meet the exacting diagnostic criteria of systems such as DSM-5, which require the presence of large numbers of uncommon medically unexplained symptoms. Conditions such as ICD-11 bodily distress disorder (formerly neurasthenia and fatigue syndromes) are more prevalent in both community and clinical populations, although it is not known to what extent they are over- or under-represented in older age groups. Similarly, the life course of these disorders has not been systematically studied, but clinical experience suggests that, when severe, they can be very persistent.

Older patients with somatic disorders usually come with thick notes and long histories of investigation and intervention. They may have avoided psychiatrists earlier in life and have deeply entrenched behaviours and beliefs about their symptoms that are difficult to challenge. The onset of genuine physical ill health in old age complicates matters still further.

In contrast to the somatiser, the hypochondriac is concerned that they might be ill, and they usually present to services looking for investigation rather than treatment. Hypochondriasis arising in old age is usually secondary to another disorder, such as depression.

Management of Neurotic Disorders in Old Age

Within health services, most neurotic disorders in older patients are encountered in primary care and the general hospital, and this is where they should be managed, at least in the first instance. Old age psychiatry services are usually not resourced to provide for this group, except in the more severe and intractable cases. However, they are an important source of education and support to colleagues in other clinical and residential settings; this can be offered when it becomes apparent from referrals for specialist help that they are having difficulty identifying or dealing with certain problems. If and as specialist old age liaison-consultation services develop further, there will be more opportunities to offer training and supervision to staff working in acute medical units.

Psychological Approaches

Cognitive Behaviour Therapy (CBT)

Despite the fact that interventions such as supportive therapy and CBT are of proven efficacy for a wide range of neurotic disorders in adults, and associated with fewer adverse side effects than drug treatments, their use with older patients has been somewhat limited. Admittedly, the evidence base for their effectiveness is smaller for older than for younger adults, but it has been shown consistently that for the relatively high-functioning young-old (usually) female patient with GAD, both supportive therapy and CBT are superior to staying on a waiting list, with an average effect size of 0.55. Positive results with CBT have also been reported for older patients with depression, panic and phobias. Such patients' limited access to these forms of treatment is likely due to scarcity of resources (trained therapists) and ageism within services. Whatever resources are allocated by health services for particular psychological treatments, these should be distributed equitably across all age groups, unless there is a good evidence to indicate that this is not cost-effective.

CBT embraces a range of educational, cognitive and behavioural therapeutic techniques that, while theoretically distinct, are usually deployed in combination to modify the problematic thinking and behaviour that occur in neurotic disorders. The cognitive component addresses the negative thoughts, false attributions and cognitive distortions that distort the patient's perception of themselves, the world and the future, and which underlie and drive their coping style and behaviour. The behavioural component of CBT engages more directly with these behaviours, using concepts such as conditioning, avoidance and reinforcement derived from learning theory. A common theme underpinning both the cognitive and the behavioural elements of the therapy is the encouragement of greater self-control of thoughts, feelings and behaviour. Both approaches require the detailed assessment of the patient, which may involve diary-keeping, and the use of standardised self-report measures such as the Beck Depression Inventory, the Automatic Thought Questionnaire and the Dysfunctional Attitude Scale. A detailed individual treatment plan is then formulated, based on the findings of the assessment. This plan will involve both sessions engaged in specific tasks with the therapist, and 'homework' to build on the progress made. In patients with anxiety symptoms, these will be addressed with psychoeducation and relaxation training.

In older patients, the assessment will also need to include factors such as physical ill health and disability, sensory loss and cognitive impairment. While none of these is a contraindication to CBT per se, they may place limits on what can be achieved, or require modifications to standard procedures. Presumably, there are some individuals, for example those with severe dysmnesia, with whom little can be achieved; however, it is not yet clear where the limits to the efficacy of CBT lie in this age group. Another issue requiring further study in older patients is the use of individual versus group CBT. Group treatment has the advantage of being more cost-effective, and it can harness useful peer-group support to improve outcomes. However, problems can arise if the group is too heterogeneous and lacks important shared experiences; careful selection and preparation of patients is important, but can be time-consuming and difficult. More task-based interventions, such as anxiety management and relaxation training, may be easier to deliver effectively in a group context.

Psychodynamic Therapy

For a long time, psychoanalysts and other psychodynamically oriented psychotherapists followed Freud in his belief that 'near or above the age of 50 the elasticity of the mental processes, on which treatment depends, is as a rule lacking – old people are no longer educable'. In the past 40 years however, a number of authors have become interested in the psychodynamics of the ageing process, and the role of the therapist in helping individuals who have difficulty adjusting to this. The most important theme discussed in this literature is that of loss – of health, status, family and friends, sexual vigour, life – and the various difficult and destructive ways that some individuals respond to this as they grow old. These include anxiety, depression, anger, envy, acting out, passive aggression and somatisation, all of which are commonly encountered in the older patients seen by health and social care services.

How then should psychodynamically oriented therapists contribute to the treatment and care of these patients? There will never be enough such therapists available or willing to offer individual treatment to all who might benefit, so this limited expertise needs to be deployed carefully. There may be a few particularly difficult, dangerous and resource-intensive patients who need to be taken on for long-term individual or group therapy, but therapists probably will have the greatest impact through the education and supervision of other health professionals, all of whom need some understanding of psychodynamics, defence mechanisms (particularly projection and projective identification) and transference/countertransference issues in order to work effectively with this group. They can also help health professionals to reflect on the dynamics that operate within their team, and between their service and other agencies in the wider world. There is now widespread recognition that the provision of reflective practice or other staff support groups can be most useful for all health services.

Drug Treatments

Despite the efficacy and better safety profile of psychological interventions such as CBT, many older patients with anxiety are treated with drugs. This is surprising, given that the evidence base is still extremely limited, and most of our practice is based on the literature on younger adults, and on clinical experience and anecdote. Rational prescribing should adhere to the following principles:

1. Thorough assessment and accurate diagnosis are the necessary foundations of any effective management plan. Too often in modern fast-throughput health services, drug treatment is merely a convenient way of avoiding a more painstaking assessment of patients' symptoms and circumstances.

2. Consider the available non-pharmacological alternatives, in particular CBT and environmental interventions. Medication is only one part of a comprehensive plan that also includes psychological and social interventions such as CBT, patient education, lifestyle advice, bibliotherapy and supportive counselling. In the absence of compelling evidence for a particular treatment, patient preference and choice are important considerations.

3. 'Start low and go slow.' Many of the drugs used in the management of anxiety are less efficiently metabolised and eliminated in older patients.

4. Set clear goals for the treatment at the outset. These might include symptom relief without sedation; improvement in sleep, freedom from physical and cognitive side effects, and avoidance of physical dependence and drug interactions. These goals should be agreed with the patient, to facilitate discontinuation if they are not achieved.

5. Give an adequate trial of treatment. Some drugs, for example antidepressants, take some weeks to have their full effect.

6. At the outset, decide how long a course of anxiolytic drug treatment will be. Many patients end up with repeat prescriptions merely because no thought has been given as to whether the drug is still needed.

7. Be aware of the possible adverse consequences of treatment, for example unpleasant or risky side effects, drug interactions, potential for dependency and abuse and toxicity in overdose.

Drug Treatment of Specific Disorders

Acute Anxiety Reactions

An anxious response to stressful events is not uncommon at any age. In some circumstances (e.g. before a medical or dental procedure), it may be appropriate to manage this with a short course of a short-acting benzodiazepine (e.g. oxazepam, lorazepam; see later in the chapter), in addition to reassurance and explanation. It is likely that much of what is labelled 'agitation' in individuals with severe dementia is in fact acute anxiety, and if drug treatment is required, a benzodiazepine may be safer and more effective than a neuroleptic (see Chapter 5).

Generalised Anxiety Disorder (GAD)

At all ages, benzodiazepines are the most frequently prescribed drug in the management of GAD; in both younger and older patients, the limited available evidence indicates they are better than placebo. Antidepressant drugs, such as paroxetine and venlafaxine, are effective anxiolytics in younger patients with GAD. Treatment with an antidepressant should always be considered in older GAD patients with comorbid depressive symptoms. For a more detailed account of antidepressant treatment in this age group, see Chapter 7.

The acute phase of treatment of GAD lasts a few weeks, and the aim is resolution of symptoms. The chronic phase aims to optimise the use of medication with minimal side effects. In older patients, short-acting benzodiazepines should be used to avoid drug accumulation and side effects such as daytime drowsiness, cognitive impairment, ataxia, fatigue, paradoxical reactions and respiratory depression. Patients develop tolerance to the effects of benzodiazepines, so they should not be used for long-term treatment; in these circumstances, an anxiolytic antidepressant or buspirone is preferable. However, because of the delayed onset of action of the antidepressants and buspirone, initial short-term treatment with a benzodiazepine may be necessary. Benzodiazepines may cause rebound anxiety on dose reduction or withdrawal.

Panic Disorder

The lack of evidence regarding treatment of panic disorder in late life is probably a consequence of its relative rarity in this population. Selective serotonin reuptake inhibitors (SSRIs) are the drugs of first choice for panic attacks and panic disorder in younger adults. Some patients with panic disorder experience feelings of increased anxiety when beginning treatment with an SSRI. For that reason, the initial dose should be lower than that usually prescribed to patients with depression. Panic does not respond to SSRI treatment for at least 4 weeks, and a full response may take 8–12 weeks. The initial phase of treatment may be covered by the addition of a short course of a short-acting benzodiazepine.

Obsessive-Compulsive Disorder (OCD)

OCD is usually treated with a combination of drugs and CBT. Clomipramine is the most extensively studied treatment for OCD, but significant anticholinergic and antihistaminic side effects limit its usefulness in older patients. In this age group, the drug of first choice would be an SSRI. The effective dose for the treatment of OCD with SSRIs tends to be higher than that required for depression, and the time taken to respond is typically much longer, at about 18 weeks. Long-term therapy is required, as discontinuation of medication usually leads to relapse. Evidence for the use of other drugs in OCD is very limited, although augmentation of SSRI treatment with either buspirone or lithium may be effective. Drug treatment appears to be more effective for obsessional thoughts than for compulsive behaviours.

Phobic Disorders

As in younger patients, CBT is the treatment of choice for phobic disorders in old age, and drugs have a relatively minor role to play.

Post-traumatic Stress Disorder

SSRIs such as paroxetine and sertraline are of benefit in the treatment of PTSD in younger adults.

Somatic Symptom Disorders

There are no studies of any form of treatment in older patients. In younger adults, antidepressants do not appear to be effective in chronic fatigue, but they may help patients with fibromyalgia and chronic pain.

PERSONALITY DISORDERS

Introduction

Personality and its disorders in old age have been little studied, either in clinical groups or in the general population. It is commonly supposed that personality changes with age, but most models of personality development predict a stable construct after the formative influences of early life have had their effect. The limited evidence from a few longitudinal studies supports the notion that personality remains relatively stable throughout adult life, apart perhaps from some increase in introversion with age. It may be that the impression of change given by cross-sectional studies is due to cohort effects. The personalities and attitudes of today's older generation were formed at a very different time and in a very different culture from today's young adults.

What may change with age is not so much one's particular cluster of personality traits, but the specific advantages and vulnerabilities they may confer at different times of life. Indeed, personality and coping styles are likely to be important factors (along with others, such as health, income, education) determining how an individual adjusts to the various challenges of growing up and growing old. How one should adapt to old age, and just what constitutes 'successful ageing' are questions that tend to receive rather value-laden responses from writers and researchers, with much debate revolving around whether it is more appropriate to remain active or to disengage from the world and its cares. In general, it appears that a good quality of life in old age is associated with maintaining one's interests and social networks, but there is still much we do not know about personality and adjustment to ageing, and it is likely that individuals will differ considerably in what kind of coping strategies and psychological defences work best for them. There are some coping styles that do appear to be associated with poor adjustment to old age, however. In particular, rigid and narcissistic individuals have great difficulty in accepting the limitations, disappointments and petty humiliations of ageing, and may respond by either angrily demanding or refusing the support of others. In the context of depression, such traits are an important risk factor for self-harm and suicide in old age.

Personality disorders are characterised by pervasive, enduring, extreme and inflexible patterns of behaviour in response to a wide range of personal and social situations. They are usually, but not always, associated with subjective distress and impairment of functioning. In the modern psychiatric classifications, specific categories of personality disorder are described and defined (see Table 9.2); these are grouped into four clusters. This approach has brought a degree of clarity and rigour to a complex field, but there are a number of important shortcomings. As with the neurotic disorders, the imposition of categorical diagnoses onto what are essentially dimensional constructs leads to problems such as how to classify individuals who do not fully meet diagnostic criteria for one or more disorders but who are nevertheless clearly disturbed. The relationship between personality and other disorders is not

Table 9.2 Current classifications of personality disorders

ICD-11 PERSONALITY DISORDERS AND RELATED TRAITS	DSM-5 PERSONALITY DISORDERS
	Cluster A
	301.0 Paranoid
ICD-11 abolished all specific types	301.20 Schizoid
of PD described in ICD-10, replacing	301.22 Schizotypal
them with a definition of PD, a dimension	
of severity, a description of specific traits	*Cluster B*
and the introduction of the concept of	301.7 Antisocial
personality difficulty	301.83 Borderline
	301.50 Histrionic
	301.81 Narcissistic
	Cluster C
	301.82 Avoidant
	301.6 Dependent
	301.4 Obsessive-compulsive
	Other Personality Disorders
	301.1 Personality change due to a
	medical condition
	301.89 Other specified PD
	301.9 Unspecified PD
F62: *Enduring personality changes, not*	
attributable to brain damage and disease	
.0: After catastrophic experience	
.1: After psychiatric illness	
.2: Other	
.3: Unspecified	

always clear; for example, where does chronic anxiety belong? With regard to older patients, an important problem is that the diagnostic criteria do not take any account of age-related issues that may influence the presentation of personality disorder, such as physical illness or disability; cognitive impairment; and changes in social role and functioning (e.g. retirement, lack of social support). As a result, some personality disorders may be inappropriately over- or under-diagnosed in this age group. Another problem with older patients is that it may be difficult to obtain a history of problems dating back to childhood and early adulthood.

There have been no longitudinal studies that have followed patients with the full range of personality disorders into old age, but cross-sectional studies using standardised questionnaires and classifications show a different profile of personality disorders at different ages. In younger patients, the most prevalent DSM personality disorders are antisocial, borderline and passive-aggressive, whereas in older patients paranoid, schizoid and anankastic disorders are more common. It has been proposed that personality disorders may divide into those that are 'immature' (mostly Cluster B) and those that are 'mature' (mostly Cluster A). The mature disorders tend to be more stable with increasing age, whereas the immature disorders appear to ameliorate over time. Long-term follow-up studies of antisocial and borderline personality support this maturation hypothesis. A key element of this maturation may be a reduction in impulsivity and aggression with age, as the disorders of young adulthood are all characterised by lability of affect and behaviour. Surveys of various clinical populations agree that DSM personality disorders become less common with age. This may be because the immature disorders are declining, but it is also possible that current diagnostic systems are not very good at capturing personality disorder as it is manifest in old age.

Personality Disorder and Psychiatric Disorder

Both dysfunctional personality traits and more severe personality disorders are associated with other psychiatric disorders, but the nature of this relationship is complex and multifactorial. There are problems with accurately determining pre-morbid personality during and after an episode of psychiatric disorder, but research does indicate that depressed and anxious patients have higher rates of pre-morbid personality dysfunction. This is more pronounced in younger than older patients, with older patients more likely to have Cluster C (anxious-fearful) criteria. Although evidence is limited, there are indications that it is those older patients with an onset of depression in early life that show the highest rates of pre-morbid personality dysfunction.

With regard to late onset schizophrenia, this is associated with higher rates of Cluster A personality disorders, although it is sometimes difficult in practice to distinguish between these disorders and the prodromal phase of the schizophrenia (see Chapter 8).

An issue of some clinical importance is the extent to which comorbid personality dysfunction influences the outcome of an episode of psychiatric disorder. Evidence is limited, suggesting that while there may not be an effect on short-term outcome, rates of relapse and service use in the longer term are more frequent. Dependent traits may be associated with more chronic forms of depression. Specific adverse outcomes, such as deliberate self-harm and suicide, are associated with Cluster C traits in late life.

Personality and Organic Brain Disorders

This is another challenge to the current classifications and methods of assessment. Behaviour change in the context of disorders such as dementia or stroke is well-recognised, particularly if the frontal lobes are involved, and recognising and managing this is an important part of the care of these patients. However, it is often not clear to what extent these changes in behaviour are secondary to cognitive impairment, or to the coarsening or exaggeration of pre-morbid personality traits. The assessment of personality in the context of cognitive impairment is hard, and usually requires informants; their judgements, however, have been found to be unreliable.

Management of Personality Disorders in Old Age

Personality disorders at all ages have traditionally been deemed untreatable, with management consisting of structural and environmental interventions to limit their adverse consequences. However, an evidence base is developing, at least in younger adults, for the efficacy of some forms of psychological intervention in these disorders, notably psycho-dynamic and cognitive therapies (see earlier in the chapter). Unfortunately, most of the trials to date have been in patients with borderline and antisocial personality disorders, not in the Cluster A and C conditions more commonly encountered in late life. There is no evidence to support the use of drug treatments for personality disorders in older patients; in the individual case, the presence or absence of a comorbid Axis I disorder would be the best guide to appropriate pharmacotherapy.

In the absence of evidence, what is to be done? There should be careful assessment, diagnosis and treatment of any underlying psychiatric disorders. What on first acquaintance appear to be dysfunctional personality traits may turn out to be symptoms of a chronic and inadequately treated affective disorder. The role, if any, of organic brain disease also needs to be determined. Physical illness and disability need to be assessed and their management optimised. At this point there needs to be a realistic setting of goals, agreed if possible with the patient and their family. Depending upon what these goals are, a number of interventions may then be tried, such as cognitive-behavioural strategies to target specific behaviours (e.g. deliberate self-harm or substance abuse); grief work; life review; and environmental adaptations up to and including institutionalisation to counter isolation and self-neglect.

Further Reading

Article

Flint, A. (2005). Generalised anxiety disorder in elderly patients: epidemiology, diagnosis and treatment options. *Drugs and Aging*, 22, 101–114. doi: 10.2165/00002512-200522020-00002.

Good overview from a leading expert.

Ramos, A. and Stanley, M. A. (2020). Anxiety disorders in late life. *Clinics in Geriatric Medicine*, 36, 237–246. doi: 10.1016/j.cger.2019.11.005

Comprehensive, contemporary review article.

Book chapters

Byrne, G. (2020). Anxiety disorders in older people. In T. Dening, A. Thomas, R. Stewart and J.-P. Taylor (eds.). *The Oxford Textbook of Old Age Psychiatry 3rd Edition*, Oxford: Oxford University Press, pp 655–670.

A very good summary of current knowledge written by a world leader in the field.

Woods, B. and Windle, G. (2020). The effects of ageing on personality. In T. Dening, A. Thomas, R. Stewart and J.-P. Taylor (eds.). *The Oxford Textbook of Old Age Psychiatry 3rd Edition*, Oxford: Oxford University Press, pp 695–704.

Everything you always wanted to know about personality and ageing.

Books

Evans, S. and Garner, J. (2020). *Talking over the Years: a Handbook of Dynamic Psychotherapy with Older Adults*. London: Brunner-Routledge.

An excellent description of the psychodynamic approach to older adults.

Goldberg, D. and Huxley, P. (1992). *Common Mental Disorders: a Biopyschosocial Model*. London: Routledge.

An important and influential book which outlines the nature, significance and treatability of neurotic disorders in clear, straightforward prose.

Chapter 10

Substance Abuse and Iatrogenesis in Late Life

Introduction

Substance abuse in late life is under-recognised as a problem and neglected as a significant risk factor in the development of some mental disorders in this population. Research in this area is sparse.

Alcohol abuse is more prevalent than any other substance abuse in the elderly, but alcohol use disorders have not had adequate attention in their recognition and management.

There is a complex relationship between alcohol consumption and the physical and mental health of older adults, whose age-related physiological function alterations will change this relationship as compared with young adults. The social environments of the elderly generally are different from those of the young and tend to change over time, which will have an impact upon their psychosocial stability and patterns of alcohol use.

Health professionals working with this population require special alertness in their clinical work so as not to miss identifying these syndromes and to provide prompt and effective assistance to older people who have 'hidden' alcohol use or substance use disorders.

Alcohol Use Disorders

Prevalence

There are very few well-constructed epidemiological studies that have examined alcohol use and abuse among representative aged populations. Those that are available have methodological issues involving definitions, measurements and confounding factors that require attention when interpreting the data.

Most studies express self-reports in a number of drinks or drinking days or number of drinks per day. In the quantity/frequency approach, subjects are asked to report what they drink on different days using a 'standard drink' as a reference. The results are then expressed as average number of drinks (or units) per day, per week and so on. However, this approach will not account for some patterns of drinking such as binge drinking, past heavy consumption with current lower consumption or cumulative alcohol consumption over a lifetime.

In Australia, a standard drink is defined as 10 g of alcohol, which is found in 375 ml of light beer or 285 ml of regular strength beer, 30 ml of spirits, 90–120 ml of wine. European studies use 8 g as a standard drink, while in the United States it is 0.5 ounces (13 g) of alcohol, which is equivalent to 1.5 ounces (45 ml) of sprits, 5 ounces (150 ml) of wine and 12 ounces (360 ml) of beer.

In the United States, light to moderate drinking is one to two drinks per day, whereas in the Rotterdam Health Study, one to three drinks per day is the benchmark; it is one to six drinks per day in the Cardiovascular Health Study!

Community surveys report a range of alcohol abuse prevalence rates from 1 per cent of women (Liverpool) and 27 per cent of men (Newcastle-upon-Tyne,) in the United Kingdom to 2 per cent of women and 22 per cent of men in the United States. In treatment settings, the alcohol abuse prevalence rate ranges from a low of 6.5 per cent (Nottingham, UK), 7.5 per cent (Adelaide, Australia) of psychogeriatric inpatients to a high of 21 per cent in a general hospital inpatient study from Baltimore, USA.

However, most community studies do report a decline in alcohol consumption with increasing age in cross-sectional studies. Whether this is due to a true decrease or whether it reflects differences in cohort effects, increased physiological effects per drink, medical problems which impact on accessibility and/or desirability of alcohol, aspects of the changing social and domestic lifestyle of the elderly or simply the likelihood that heavy drinkers die young is opaque.

Metabolism of Alcohol in Late Life

With increasing age, physiological changes alter the metabolism of all substances, including alcohol. Changes in absorption, plasma binding and renal excretion and decreased body water, all lead to higher blood alcohol concentrations. Such physiological changes, together with altered metabolism, are likely to result in the occurrence of more damage for the same level of intake compared with younger people. Associated with this are the altered effects of alcohol in the elderly, such as increased functional impairment with the same blood levels, decreased euphoric effects and decreased capacity to develop tolerance. Alcohol also will aggravate medical and psychiatric diseases and disorders, increase cognitive impairment and reduce sensory and motor capacity.

Such increases in the damaging effects of alcohol use in the elderly need to be factored in when assessing the alcohol intake by older adults.

Health-Related Effects of Excessive Consumption of Alcohol in the Elderly

While the major effects of excess alcohol consumption overlaps that of younger adults, there are special considerations applying to the elderly. Heavy intake (five or more drinks daily) is associated with a quadrupled risk of developing cognitive impairment. A problematic drinking history quite substantially increases the risk of depression, psychiatric illnesses and memory problems.

While only 20 per cent of studies report harm associated with increased alcohol exposure, the physician should be alert for individuals whose increased alcohol intake may be associated with (if not causal for) risk of falls and fractures, decreased functional ability, driving impairment, drug interaction and delirium.

Although heavy alcohol consumption is an established risk for the development of dementia, recent population studies including the Rotterdam Study, the Copenhagen City Heart Study and the Cardiovascular Health Study, have suggested, however, that light to moderate drinking (one to three drinks per day – Rotterdam Study, one to six drinks per day – Cardiovascular Health Study) is associated with a lower risk for dementia. The

Copenhagen City Heart Study showed no relationship between alcohol intake and the risk of dementia. Exclusive wine drinkers seem to have a lower risk of developing dementia. Such a conclusion was also reached in a Stockholm Study.

The relationship between alcohol dependence and suicide in a Swedish study revealed that a history of alcohol dependence was observed in 35 per cent of elderly men and 18 per cent in elderly woman who died by suicide. On the other hand, in the control group, 2 per cent of men and 1 per cent of women had alcohol dependence or misuse. The odds ratio was calculated to be 18-fold in men with an alcohol disorder and 9.5-fold in women. Alcohol use disorder is an independent risk factor for predicting suicide in late life and is associated with non-violent methods in the final act.

Late Onset Alcoholism

A significant proportion of alcohol abusers take up heavy drinking in old age. The term 'late onset alcoholism' refers to those whose previous 'normal' drinking habits become heavy and to previous non-drinkers who develop alcohol abuse in late life.

The physical, mental and environment effects of ageing seem to be related to this change from normal to pathological alcohol intake. Reactive life factors such as bereavement, retirement, loneliness, physical infirmity and relationship stress are indicators of risk.

This concept, however, is not universally accepted as most elderly people do not drink excessively despite the 'stresses of ageing', and not all late onset drinkers attribute such stresses as reasons for their drinking.

It is likely that a small group of older people may develop drinking problems for the first time in late life when they adversely react to negative life events such as bereavement and retirement. The possibility of better prognosis and response to intervention in restoring their life and psychological balance should lead to some level of optimism when these patients are identified.

Management of Alcohol Problems in Late Life

The first step in management begins with identification of the problem. Some special and personal changes provide suggestive pointers which should raise the clinician's suspicions. Self-neglect is associated with cognitive decline; evidence of poor nutrition; unexplained falls, accidents, injuries; unstable and poorly controlled physical illness (diabetes, hypertension); failure to keep appointments and poor compliance with treatment; increasing conflict with family members; the persistence of gastrointestinal problems; and unexplained delirium during hospitalisation for medical treatment are all possible pointers to the presence of alcohol abuse.

When alcohol abuse is suspected in the older patient, a detailed history of alcohol intake needs to be checked with family members and a visit to the home should be scheduled. During this visit there should be inspection to check for stacks of empty bottles in the back garden or the rubbish bins, any stock of alcohol in cupboards and pantries and any evidence of neglect of the home should be noted.

Should detoxification be required, this must be done in hospital, particularly if the patient is at risk of life-threatening sequelae of intoxication, accidental events or severe risk to existing medical illness. During detoxification it will be necessary to be alert for the withdrawal symptoms of *delirium tremens,* including tremor, insomnia, sweating, nausea or vomiting, transient frightening visual, auditory or tactile hallucinations, psychomotor hyperactivity, severe anxiety and fear, autonomic hyperactivity and withdrawal seizures.

Time-limited use of short-acting benzodiazepines can be useful in treatment of symptoms of alcohol withdrawal. Thiamine (both intravenous and oral), with other vitamin supplements, is always useful as most alcohol abusers are nutritionally impaired. The use of novel antipsychotics with sedating properties in low doses may be required to manage frightening hallucinations, although these drugs can lower the fit threshold. General supportive care aimed towards restoration of physiological and psychological balance should be undertaken during detoxification.

After detoxification, the management will include a thorough assessment of both the physical and psychosocial status of the patient. In particular, the repertoire of psychological and personality strengths and resilience in the history of the patient should be utilised. Such factors are useful tools to be deployed in psychotherapeutic interventions to follow. The strength, extent and availability of family support will also be assessed. Identifying and treating medical and psychiatric comorbidity must be undertaken thoroughly. Depression, hypertension and cardiovascular diseases; painful conditions, such as arthritis; and late onset diabetes, all will need to be investigated and treated energetically, as these frequently contribute to the general well-being of the patient, and management can remove some of the contributing effects of disability secondary to alcohol overuse.

Psychotherapeutic interventions using such strategies as Cognitive Behavioural Therapy, Interpersonal Psychotherapy, or Marital/Family therapy as indicated will be the mainstay of resolving basic underlying drives in the patient's motivation to continue alcohol abuse.

The adjunctive contribution of spiritual support in patients who have a past history of spiritual activities, or who wish to embark on a new spiritual direction, should always be included in a holistic programme management. As in all areas of old age psychiatry, the multidisciplinary model involving all healthcare professionals – physiotherapy, occupational therapy, nursing, dietician, podiatrist, speech pathologist – in the care of these patients can contribute to the success of treatment. Such professionals may enhance quality of life and thus add positive meaning to counter the urge to return to (ab)using alcohol.

Outcome

Although existing studies tend to be pessimistic regarding interventions, with about one in seven having good outcomes, those who continue in treatment programmes are more likely to be successful. Late onset drinkers are often socially isolated, widowed yet highly motivated. An expansion of social networks is associated with improvement and with completion of therapy. Keeping the patient in a treatment programme by enhancing their expectations and motivations, thus providing an expanded social network and support, may lead to a better outcome.

Other Substance Abuse Disorders and Iatrogenesis

Illicit Substances

Past generations of older people were not much given to the abuse of illicit substances available to younger adults. However, as the 'baby boomers' have entered old age, an increasing number who used illicit substances in their youth either continue or resume in old age. This generation bring with them new challenges and open up new varieties of mental health problems, not much encountered in routine old age psychiatry practice until recent times.

Health professionals should be vigilant in identifying those who may use illicit drugs either as a lifestyle habit or who abuse them as a substitute for psychosocial support in their old age.

Prescribed Medications – Iatrogenesis

A serious current problem in substance abuse is that of prescribed dependency promoting medications.

The entry of benzodiazepines into the medical world was an initial boon as they displaced the barbiturate dependence problem, which was quite serious in the 1950s and 1960s, and accompanied by significant risk of accidental, fatal overdose. Members of the current generation of older people sometimes were switched from barbiturates to benzodiazepines for the treatment of anxiety and insomnia, though there are very few of these still around, but many others had benzodiazepine drugs initiated de novo and continued to receive prescriptions for many years thereafter. Some continue on the same dosage into old age with little harm. However, dependence occurs in some people who after reaching old age begin to use benzodiazepines to manage emotional and psychological distress, as well as for depression and early cognitive change, while others continue an earlier pattern of dependence or abuse into their later years. Such dependence has serious health consequences, which may include multiple falls and fractures, resulting in disability and even death. Many studies have identified the role of benzodiazepine hypnotics (even in the non-dependent elderly) as a risk factor for falls and fractures, especially in residential care and notably among those with comorbid dementia. Excessive sedation encourages immobility and may increase the risk of hypostatic pneumonia, aggravate joint pathology and reduce exposure to sunlight with resultant vitamin deficiencies and consequent bone disorders. The quality of life impacts of overuse of benzodiazepines among elderly people are of major medical and ethical concern.

If benzodiazepines are indicated at all for older adults, they must be used in the lowest possible dose for the shortest period of time and be reviewed regularly to see if the dosage can be reduced or be ceased.

Health professionals working in residential care should be alert to the harmful effects of benzodiazepine overuse and exercise due care in preventing such problems from developing. The use of benzodiazepines for 'behavioural control' is at best inappropriate and at worst may represent professional misconduct. Virtually all elderly people who experienced problems of benzodiazepine toxicity, withdrawal symptoms or other adverse effects originally started to take them on medical advice. Despite the fact that the elderly are the most vulnerable members of the population to the adverse effects of benzodiazepines, they continue to be more likely to be prescribed these drugs than are younger adults, though in most places prescription rates have declined in recent years. Prevention is better than cure and in this case the solution to the problem lies in medical practitioners initiating the prescription of these drugs less often and less readily, especially to elderly patients.

Conclusion

Healthcare workers who see older adults should be alert to the misuse and abuse of alcohol and prescribed substances as well as illicit substances. Comprehensive management using a biopsychosocial spiritual approach can help some old people who misuse and abuse such substances. Alertness in identifying pointers to substance misuse and abuse requires constant vigilance. A sensitive and caring questioning of the older patient in these areas is necessary and should always be part of history taking and examination as well as a vital component of any home visits.

Multidisciplinary and multi-modal treatments should be energetically and optimistically applied to ensure the best possible, and improved, quality of life. In the endeavour to assist older people affected by substance abuse, the professional's strongest ally will usually be the patient's family.

Further Reading

Articles

Ganguli, M., Vanderbilt, J., Saxton, J. A., Shen, C. and Dodge H. H. (2005). Alcohol consumption and cognitive function in late life. *Neurology*, 65, 1210–1217. doi: 10.1212/01.wnl.0000180520.35181.24.

Highlights the potential for harm associated with late life alcohol abuse.

Graham, K., Carver V. and Brett, P. J. (1996). Alcohol and drug use by older women: result of a national survey. *Canadian Journal of Ageing*, 14, 769–791. doi: 10.1017/S0714980800016457.

A good study giving plausible prevalence figures.

Graham K., Clarke C., Bors C., Carver V., Dolinski L., Smyth C. and Harrison S. (1996). Addictive behaviour of older adults. *Addictive Behaviour*, 21, 331–348. doi: 10.1016/0306-4603(95)00065-8.

An account of the phenomenon of addiction in late life with regard to prescribed substances as well as licit and illicit drugs of abuse.

Patterson, T. L. and Jeste, D. V. (1999). The potential impact of the baby-boomer generation on substance abuse amongst elderly persons. *Psychiatric Services*, 50, 1184–1188. doi: 10.1176/ps.50.9.1184.

Highlights the possible effects of the maturation of the post-war generation on substance abuse patterns.

Rigler, S. K. (2000). Alcoholism in the elderly. *American Family Physician*, 61, 1710–1766.

Focuses on the more severe end of the alcohol abuse spectrum in late life.

Ticehurst, S. (1990). Alcohol in the elderly. *Australian and New Zealand Journal of Psychiatry*, 24, 252–260. doi: 10.3109/00048679009077690.

This clear and thorough article is still pertinent 31 years after it was written.

Whelan, G. (2003). Alcohol: a much neglected risk factor in elderly mental disorders. *Current Opinion in Psychiatry*, 1, 609–614. doi: 10.1097/00001504-200311000-00002.

Evidence-based overview.

Book chapter

Gambert, S. and Albrecht III, C. (2005). Chapter 63. In J. L. Lewinson, P. Ruiz and R. Millman (eds.). *Substance Abuse: a Comphrensive Textbook 4th Edition*, Baltimore: Williams & Wilkins, pp. 1038–1048.

Rao, T. and Jones, K. (2020). Alcohol and substance abuse. In: T. Dening, A. Thomas, R. Stewart and J.-P. Taylor (eds.). *The Oxford Textbook of Old Age Psychiatry 3rd Edition,* Oxford: Oxford University Press, pp 713–734.

Both these chapters provide thorough, evidence-based overviews.

Services for Older Patients with Psychiatric Disorders

Brief Historical Notes

The emergence of dedicated services for older people with mental disorders is a fairly recent phenomenon in health services around the world. Until the 1950s, aged people with severe mental disorders were treated and housed in large mental hospitals located away from the general community.

In the 1950s, important research into the mental disorders of late life began in the United Kingdom. This work highlighted the fact that these disorders are important entities deserving special attention. Reports of a series of scandals stirred policymakers to consider new management models. This, in conjunction with a more positive attitude towards older people, derived from the research of Roth, Kiloh, Kay, Blessed, Bergman, Corsellis, Post and others combined to lead to a more enlightened approach. In the United States, Butler at the Institute of Mental Health led research in human ageing, whilst in 1959, the World Health Organisation convened the first meeting of its expert committee on the mental health of the aged, which was followed by a Conference on 'Mental Disorders in the Aged' by the World Psychiatric Association in 1965.

From the 1960s, in Britain and North America, a process of development of special attention towards older people with mental disorders focused on moving those with serious mental illnesses out of the large mental hospitals into community settings. By the 1980s, especially in the United Kingdom, emerging specialist services for old people came into being, underpinned by the principles of comprehensive old age psychiatry services – flexibility, responsiveness, availability, un-hierarchical use of staff, domiciliary assessment and willingness to collaborate with other services and agencies.

This British model was championed by Tom Arie, who through the British Council courses in psychogeriatrics promulgated it to other parts of the world, including Canada, Australia, Continental Europe, Scandinavia, South Africa and Hong Kong. Many of the old age psychiatry services in developed countries around the world adapted this 'Arie Model' to suit local conditions. The model aimed to have a global perspective, to include residential homes, to respect the roles of allied health and nursing staff, highlight the importance of liaison work in general hospitals and to enhance interdisciplinary relations, especially working with the primary health system.

International Consensus Model on Organisations of Care

The influence of the British leaders in the early development of psychogeriatric services (Arie, Pitt, Post, Jolley) led to the establishment of services to older people, which included comprehensive assessment (preferably at the person's locale), and served the population of potential patients in a local community.

Central to this is the multidisciplinary psychogeriatric team with a consultant psychiatrist, committed to old people, leading such a team which includes nurses, social workers, occupational therapists, psychologists (clinical and/or neuropsychologists) and other health professionals such as physiotherapists, podiatrists, dietitians, music therapists and pharmacists according to local circumstances.

By the mid-1990s, differing models of service delivery were evolving, especially in the United Kingdom, the United States, Australia and Continental Europe and an international consensus was seen to be necessary to establish what could be considered as core international best practice.

To achieve this, the late Jean Wertheimer of Lausanne, Switzerland, as the Chair of the World Psychiatric Association Section of Geriatric Psychiatry, took the initiative in 1997 in organising a very successful Consensus Conference. Thus, a Consensus Statement with the imprimatur of the WPA and WHO with the participation of related international bodies such as IPA and other non-government organisations was prepared and published. This document provides the fundamental generic model of best practice in the organisation of care in psychogeriatric services delivery (see Further Reading section).

Specific principles of best practice in this Consensus document can be referred to as the CARITAS principles. CARITAS is the Latin word for love and care, which underpins the attitude behind the use of this acronym.

Quality care for older persons with mental health problems should be:

Comprehensive
Accessible
Responsive
Individualised
Transdisciplinary
Accountable
Systemic (Seamless)

- A *comprehensive* service should take into account all aspects of the patient's physical, psychological and social needs and wishes and be patient-centred.
- An *accessible* service is user-friendly and readily available, minimising the geographical, cultural, financial, political and linguistic obstacles to obtaining care.
- A *responsive* service is one that listens to and understands the problems brought to its attention and acts promptly and appropriately.
- An *individualised* service focuses on each person with a mental health problem in their family and community context. The planning of care must be tailored for and acceptable to the individual and family, and should aim wherever possible to maintain and support the person in their home environment.
- A *transdisciplinary* approach goes beyond traditional professional boundaries to optimise the contributions of people with a range of personal and professional skills. Such an approach also facilitates collaboration with voluntary and other agencies to provide a comprehensive range of community orientation services.
- An *accountable* service is one that accepts responsibility for assuring the quality of the service it delivers and monitors this in partnership with patients and their families. Such a service must be ethically and culturally sensitive.

- A *systemic* (seamless) approach flexibly integrates all available services to ensure continuity of care and coordinates all levels of service providers, including local, provincial and national governments and community organisations.

The transdisciplinary principle needs further explanation. In less developed countries, with few professional disciplines beyond doctor and nurse, the concepts of multidisciplinary and interdisciplinary can be difficult to apply. The Zimbabwean representative, Dr Juliet Dube-Ddebele, suggested and the Consensus group agreed that the concept principle of transdisciplinary – which has the core value of transcending disciplinary boundaries to be inclusive of all available skills from professional, lay and voluntary groups – should be promoted instead of the traditional multidisciplinary or interdisciplinary principles so valued in more developed countries.

The Multidisciplinary Team

An essential feature of the care offered by the psychiatry of old age is the multidisciplinary team which works in a transdisciplinary manner. Although the old age psychiatrist is likely to be the team leader, every attempt is made to operate in a non-hierarchical, mutually respectful and collaborative way having the welfare and quality of life of older people as a committed shared value.

Transcending disciplinary barriers can be difficult in some situations. A functional team will put such difficulties as a secondary consideration to the high priority of patient-focused decision making.

The ideal team usually consists of the following members (if available):

- The old age psychiatrist who leads the team (including family discussions), is able to think about all the relevant medical and psychosocial issues and may ultimately hold responsibility for the patient.

- The psychiatric nurse, whose role often is to provide ongoing support and monitoring of the patient, including any response to, or adverse consequences of, any treatments given. The nurse often fulfils a vital function as the patient's ally and advocate, especially if the relationship with the psychiatrist becomes strained for any reason (e.g. a need to use the involuntary treatment or detention provisions of the local Mental Health Laws).

- Occupational therapist (OT). The OT's role is to provide information about functional tasks for the patient, including the patient's ability to independently carry out activities of daily living (ADLs) such as showering, dressing, cooking, cleaning, navigational assessments and sometimes driving assessments. The OT is also responsible for lifestyle and leisure for the patients and can refer them to local activity groups.

- Social worker (SW). The SW has a role to provide information about the wider financial and legal issues. Information about power of attorneys, guardian, financial administrators, referrals to local key workers and possibly to local activity leisure groups are crucial for older adults. In addition, some countries require specific aged care assessments as a 'ticket of entry' into residential care, and the SW's role may be to organise this.

- Neuropsychologist. This person can provide detailed cognitive assessment tailored to the individual, taking into consideration the following: their age, pre-existing medical conditions that may affect this assessment (including sensory impairment), premorbid intellectual ability, and current mental state (e.g. depressive or psychotic symptoms). Strengths and weaknesses and strategies to address these and capacity assessments may also be provided by the neuropsychologist.

- Clinical psychologist. The skills of the clinical psychologist can be invaluable across a wide range of settings and patients, from the anxious person with phobias to the agitated person affected by dementia, with repetitive behaviours of concern, who resides in residential care.

- Others. Speech pathology may be required for thorough assessment of swallowing and language skills. A dietician may provide advice on nutritional intake. Trainees in all the aforementioned disciplines, especially trainee psychiatrists, often form part of the team for specified training periods and play a valuable role, while learning from experience. Last, it should be recognised that all teams have their own internal dynamics and that it is vital to foster morale and good working relationships, even when there is significant pressure of work. One should not underestimate the significance of the contributions of individuals who may organise the team football tipping competition, arrange the end of year team dinner, take up a collection for flowers to send to a team member who is sick or bereaved or leaving the team or arrange regular journal clubs and team education. Such roles are not discipline specific, tend to emerge over time in well-functioning teams and contribute to successful team functioning in ways that are not always recognised by administrators and the patients and families whom the team helps with assessment, treatment and care.

The overlap of discipline-related skills will benefit the patient by the enhancement of practical application of discipline-specific skills. For example, the nurse may apply physio-therapy and occupational therapy skills learned from them so that out of hours application of their therapeutic interventions may be continued. Knowledge and skills of good nursing practice will enhance that of the therapists during therapy activities.

Residential Care

Whilst the primary goal is to keep the older person living at home for as long as possible, residential care is a necessary option for those whose physical health, mental health and well-being are best served in the residential care environment. Formal support such as domiciliary nurses to provide personal care, delivered meals, district nurses to provide wound care, insulin and medication administration (and checking of blood glucose), transportation and respite (see section on this below) may assist in delaying the need for permanent residential care.

The quality of residential care applies to all aspects of the residential environment.

Design of the physical, built environment should be home-like, conducive to privacy, visually pleasing and provide a sense of cheerful comfort. Light and space indoors and outside space for gentle exercise, gardens for visual and olfactory pleasure should be available. The relationship of spatial areas, colours of walls and floors should be simple, safe and orientating. The use of both easily recognised symbols and words on signage should assist in orientation. Furnishings should be safe, take into account physical disability, as well as be comfortable and practical, and where possible should be consistent with the period of the older people's lives in their design. The kitchen should be open to the common space to allow for visual, auditory and olfactory contact with the residents, as well as being available to those who can use their retained food preparation skills under supervision.

While not all residents in residential care will have dementia, there are certain design principles which may reduce negative outcomes such as agitation, confusion and wandering behaviours, and increase positive outcomes such as mobility and ADLs. In Australia, the Dementia Training Study Centre developed 10 key design principles in residential care. These included the following:

1. Unobtrusively reduce risk: while safety is a priority, enabling people was also important. For example, if using a fence, ensure it is constructed from material which will allow people to see through it and enjoy the view beyond the fence.

2. Provide a human scale. Consideration of group size, as more people could lead to more distractions, potentially leading to more challenging behaviours.

3. Allow people to see and be seen. Similar to principle 1 – allowing people to see where they are in the environment, such as having a window to look outside.

4. Minimise unhealthy stimulation. This might confuse and distress those with dementia. Strategies might include painting murals to disguise exit doors.

5. Optimise helpful stimulation. Cues such as different coloured doors or a view may enable people with dementia to better find their way.

6. Support movement and engagement. Arrange the environment such that it encourages people to use the furniture or items provided. Strategies might include arranging chairs to invite and cue people to sit down.

7. Create a similar space using furniture, textures, colours and fittings to make people feel comfortable based on previous preferences.

8. Provide opportunities to be alone or to be with others.

9. Provide links with the community, such as a community garden or inviting students or young children to interact with the residents under supervision, or organising a movie night with residents and their families and friends.

10. Respond to a vision for way of life. This relates to being aware of residents' preferences and activities and encouraging them to continue with these interests, such as gardening or cooking.

The television should not be used as a 'baby-sitting' device, but utilised positively for stimulating the cognitive function of residents. Music of each resident's preference in both public and private areas will provide listening pleasure, enhance reminiscences and facilitate rhythm-related movements.

Space for leisure activities, assisted by staff members (often a recreational or leisure-lifestyle therapist), will enhance the enjoyment of daily life as will planned outings to places of interest, public festivals and entertainment.

Residential care, although having medical and nursing functions, should attempt to minimise the emphasis on these activities as much as possible to produce and maintain a more home-like environment.

Visitors (family, friends or volunteers) should be welcomed into the residential community and encouraged to bring the outside world into the facility to add value to residential care.

Other activities usually undertaken in the general community, such as shopping, hairdressing, tea and coffee houses and pets, can be brought into the facility or be made available to those residents who could leave the facility safely accompanied by staff members, relatives and friends.

The wearing of uniforms by staff is a contentious issue. Where uniform is required for identification, this should be designed to minimise the 'hospital-like' atmosphere it may evoke. If identification name badges are worn, these should be in large print and strategically placed for older people to read and recognise.

Designated quiet areas for spiritual activities, contemplation and meditation encourage those who have spiritual needs to continue to undertake their usual practices and rituals.

A deliberate emphasis on designing a sensitive and pleasing environment not only benefits residential residents directly but also engenders an atmosphere in which staff can respond with more appropriate affect and attitude.

Medical Care

As medical comorbidity is common, quality energetic medical care, usually provided by visiting primary care physicians or general practitioners (GPs), should be in place. It is recommended that if possible, all older adults have a GP who can act as the first port-of-call, has longitudinal knowledge about the patient and may act as a coordinator of care. Timely access to specialist care provides support to the GPs. As well as old age psychiatrists, other specialists the GP may refer the patients to include geriatricians and neurologists, and also relevant community allied health (e.g. OTs can visit the home to do safety and activity assessments).

Community-Based Assessment

The frontline activity of an old age psychiatry team is the place of domicile of patients and their families. All, or nearly all, assessments should occur in patients' homes. The team goes to the patient rather than the patient coming to the team. Such an approach enables the development of a better therapeutic alliance, shows that the patient and families are valued, removes obstacles to accessibility, such as mobility difficulties, and provides the opportunity to see how life is lived in each home and a more practical understanding of where support may be needed.

In countries where there is a perceived legal/liability obstacle to such an approach, advocacy to alter the legal environment should be energetically pursued through the legislature.

Respite Care

Carers of older adults with any disability can become tired and burnt-out. For those caring for people with mental illnesses, including dementia, this may be more so. Regular breaks (respite) for carers should be available, but may require forward planning and encouragement by the GP and specialist services. Carers may feel guilty that they cannot provide constant care. Options may include using home-based respite, where a substitute carer will replace the carer at home, thereby freeing up the carer to have a break. Another option is for the patient to have respite in a residential facility which may enable the carer to take lengthy (one to three weeks or more) respite at regular intervals (two to four times a year). Other useful respite options include home cleaning, home maintenance or the provision of ready-made meals. Maintaining the health and well-being of the carer is a necessary part of any quality old age psychiatry service delivery. In some countries, there are carer services which can provide support, advice and psychoeducation to carers.

Information, Advice and Public Education

The dual stigma of mental illness and ageing that is so prevalent in all countries requires constant action in de-stigmatisation by old age psychiatry services. The delivery of accurate information on both ageing and mental disorders through printed material, electronic or print media, public discussion forum and taking any opportunity to 'sell' a positive message to the general community and the health community forms a necessary part of the work of the old age psychiatry service. Collaboration with mental health organisations, NGOs and carers' groups in any activity of public education will enhance what the service does by itself.

Advocacy

Older adults may be reluctant to speak up for themselves, participate in protest marches or undertake overt political activities to make a point or demand. This may change as an activist-minded baby boomer generation and their successors become the predominant consumers of aged care services.

An old age psychiatry service with trained professionals can advocate for their patients and families to obtain the attention of policymakers who might otherwise ignore a relatively silent minority.

Equitable, accessible, affordable care services, availability of pharmaceuticals, adequate financial security, accessible and disabled friendly transport, appropriate housing and neighbourhood resources are issues that often demand the advocacy action of the service as an entity and of staff members individually. Pro-activity on behalf of older people has been a strong historical hallmark of early psychogeriatric services, especially in the United Kingdom. Such an example should be followed and expanded by all current and future services.

Spiritual and Leisure Needs

Meaningful and appropriate recreational and leisure activities contribute to quality of life of older people. Leisure, which includes gentle exercise and outdoor activities as part of pleasurable activity, has additional health benefits. The opportunity to express and practise spiritual aspects of their lives and lived experiences will contribute to their sense of peace as well as an effective preparation for their end of life directions. Helping them to resolve interpersonal and intrapersonal conflicts through spiritual means often contributes to their dying well. Each older person's spiritual needs, expressions and practices should always be respected and honoured.

What Are the Necessary Components of a Service?

To this question, irrespective of available resources, the principle of 'Surround them with care' should be central (Figure 11.1).

Resources-rich services will have more components, whereas resource-poor services will have fewer. However, rich or poor, what is available should provide an encircling support system for the patient and family. The family and local neighbourhood/community should always be considered as care components to which others are added as more resources become available. In an ideal world, the following components are considered to be the minimum acceptable:

- Community mental health teams for older persons
- Inpatient assessment and treatment

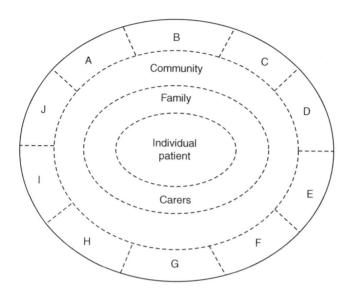

Figure 11.1 Surround them with care

- Day hospitals
- Outpatients services
- Respite care – 'in-home' or facility based
- Continuing hospital care
- Residential care
- Liaison services for general and geriatric hospitals
- Primary care collaborations
- Community and social support services
- Prevention programmes
- Educational programmes for health professionals
- Destigmatisation programmes and public education and health promotion

Innovation

Old age psychiatry services staff are usually creative and innovative people who are good problem solvers in many practical ways. This is to be encouraged, fostered and applauded.

While advancing technology can provide effective and useful solutions (e.g. Global Position Tracking, pressure pad alarm systems, key-pad-coded doors), there are many opportunities for staff to exercise their imagination aided by practical life experiences to resolve problems offered by patients and families. Some creative lateral thinking often produces very simple, affordable and satisfactory results.

Conclusion

The most effective quality service for older people with mental disorders is one which is patient- and family-centred; values and encourages staff; has an ethos of CARITAS towards older persons; uses resources effectively and wisely; and puts into effect despite any resource constraints, the principles as established by WPA/WHO Consensus Statement of 1997.

Further Reading

Articles

Hilton, C. (2005). The origins of old age psychiatry in Britain in the 1940s. *History of Psychiatry*, 16, 267–289. doi: 10.1177/ 0957154X05050075.

Excellent account of service genesis.

Hilton, C. (2015). Age inclusive services or separate old age and working age services? A historical analysis from the formative years of old age psychiatry c. 1940–1989. *BJPsych Bulletin*, 39, 90–95. doi: 10.1192/pb. bp.113.046250.

An effective refutation of the idea that older people should be dumped in with younger psychiatric patients for the provision of services (which leads to their neglect and potentially to their abuse).

Loi, S. and Hassett, A. (2011). Evolution of aged persons mental health services in Victoria: the history behind their development. *Australasian Journal on Ageing*, 30, 226–230. doi: 10.1111/j.1741-6612.2011.00529.x.

Summary of aged psychiatry services in Victoria, Australia.

Book chapters

Arie, T. (2002). The development in Britain. In J.R.M. Copeland, M.T. Abou-Saleh and D.G. Blazer (eds.). *Principles and Practice of Geriatric Psychiatry*, 2nd ed., Chichester: John Wiley, pp. 9–11.

Service-focused overview of the development of old age psychiatric services in the United Kingdom.

Snowdon, J. and Arie, T. (2005). A history of psychogeriatric services. In P. Melding, B. Draper and H. Brodaty (eds.). *Psychogeriatric Service Delivery: an International Perspective*. Oxford: Oxford University Press, pp 3–20.

Excellent summary of the history of our field.

Consensus statement

World Health Organisation. (1997). *Consensus Statement in Organization of Care in Psychiatry of the Elderly*. WHO/MSA/MNH/ 97.3. Geneva: WHO.

A prescription for service creation and implementation.

12 The Future of the Psychiatry of Old Age

Introduction

An understanding of past and current trends that bear on the mental disorders of later life informs any speculation about the future. By speculating about the future, one aims to develop a successful strategy for educating future healthcare professionals who will care for older adults. At the same time, we aim to develop an approach that will enhance our understanding of psychiatric disorders of later life. In this chapter, we summarise debates about how to 'go forward' with the full knowledge that the future is highly unpredictable (as we have seen since March 2020!). Nonetheless, it is fair to say that two major issues will continue to influence the future of the psychiatry of old age (POA).

1. POA will be profoundly affected by the future of its parent discipline, that of psychiatry, and in particular the continuing impact of neurosciences. Targeted therapeutic approaches will become increasingly important as neuroscientific understanding allows us to parse and target the aetiologic heterogeneity within neuropsychiatric syndromes. With regard to psychotherapy, the general shift towards manual-based and evidence-based short-term therapies will have a significant influence on our approach to older adults, especially those with mild cognitive impairment.

2. The second major influence will be the outcome of the ongoing debate about the future of geriatrics (geriatric medicine), a closely related discipline. Do we continue to provide age-based as opposed to needs-based or diagnosis-based services and subspecialties?

Historical Influences

In a paper written in 1994 by Dr Ken Shulman, a co-author of the first edition of this book, speculation about the future of geriatric psychiatry began with a review of historical developments that shaped the field to that point. This included the importance of leaders in mainstream psychiatry of the 1950s and 1960s (Sir Martin Roth in Newcastle and Felix Post at the Institute of Psychiatry in London) turning their attention to the study of older adults. This had the effect of legitimising the field of POA and attracting attention from mainstream trainees. Roth's paper on the 'Natural history of mental disorders' published in 1955 had its greatest impact by demonstrating the uniqueness of the three Ds: dementia, depression and delirium. Ironically, recent works covered in other chapters have demonstrated that the independence of these syndromes is not as pronounced as originally suggested by Roth. Nonetheless, that paper had a profound impact on both academic and clinical interest in POA.

Service developments in the National Health Service (NHS) of the United Kingdom made it easier to provide psychiatric services to the frail and cognitively impaired old. This in turn led pioneers in the field, like Brice Pitt and Tom Arie, to promote the importance of collaboration with the field of geriatric medicine. This has remained the primary specialty relationship for POA. The principles regarding the development of service delivery in the British NHS for geriatrics did largely inform the same approach to POA. These principles included comprehensiveness, accountability, clearly defined target populations, availability and flexibility of services with a strong focus on the community and the role of carers.

Several organisations have reflected and influenced the development of psychiatric services for older adults. In the United Kingdom, the Royal College of Psychiatrists hosted the development of an interest group for Old Age Psychiatry in 1978. This small interest group of energetic and charismatic psychiatrists went on to develop a section that now has blossomed into the Faculty of Old Age Psychiatry for the Royal College of Psychiatrists and established a credible body informing health policy and principles of service delivery. The Canadian Association of Geriatric Psychiatry has followed the direction of the Royal College of Psychiatrists by helping to inform Health Policy, especially psychiatric consultation to nursing homes. In the United States, on the other hand, the American Association of Geriatric Psychiatry (AAGP), similarly established in 1978, became an active voice within the parent American Psychiatric Association, but focused largely on academic matters and helped to stimulate a high level of clinical research in the field of geriatric psychiatry. The International Psychogeriatric Association (IPA) was subsequently established and has contributed to the dissemination of knowledge and clinical standards, and has advanced research regarding the care of older adults at a global level.

Clinical Neuroscience

The continued growth and development of clinical neurosciences may very well represent the most powerful force for change in psychiatry and in particular for POA. This involves the increasingly close and collaborative relationships with cognitive and behavioural neurology, which in turn has transformed its parent discipline of neurology over the last two decades. In 2002, Martin documented the very significant research advances in our understanding of the genetic basis of the diseases affecting the brain and central nervous system. In particular, he noted the impact of disorders such as Alzheimer's disease (AD) and Tourette's syndrome, which served as prototypes for the reasons that clinical work and research in neurology and psychiatry diverged so dramatically in the twentieth century. Defining AD by its neuropathologic hallmarks of neuronal loss, senile plaques and neurofibrillary tangles assigned this disorder to the neurologic category of disease, notwithstanding the fact that many of the features and symptoms of the disease are behavioural and psychiatric in nature. It is clear that despite its neurological substrate, a joint effort of neurologists and psychiatrists was necessary to understand how diseases of the brain not only impact upon gross motor or cognitive functions but also upon behaviour. This conceptualisation helped to blur the previously artificial categories of 'organic' and 'functional' disorders. In contrast, Gilles de la Tourette syndrome, for which there was no known neuropathological basis, remained mired in a debate about psychological versus organic causes without resolution until later years.

Historically, the division between neurology and psychiatry became more obvious after World War II, when the *Archives of Neurology and Psychiatry* published in the United States was divided into two separate journals. However, this separation became blurred as the major diseases of psychiatry, such as schizophrenia and bipolar disorder, were shown to be accompanied by significant changes in brain structure and function. Martin points out that since the 1960s, developments in neuropharmacology, and in particular the identification of neurotransmitter systems, has led to the development of biological psychiatry. Furthermore, advances in structural neuroimaging, together with increased use of functional and molecular imaging techniques, have contributed to a neuroscientific understanding of psychiatry more broadly. Martin makes reference to Winston Churchill's original characterisation of the United States and Britain as two countries separated by a common language. For neurology and psychiatry, that common language is indeed neuroscience. The Nobel Laureate, Eric Kandel argues that psychiatry can make a contribution to brain science by

> defining for biology the mental functions that need to be studied for a meaningful and sophisticated understanding of the human mind. . . . The details of the relationship between the brain and mental processes – precisely how the brain gives rise to various mental processes – is understood poorly, and only in outline. The great challenge for biology and psychiatry at this point is to delineate that relationship in terms that are satisfying to both the biologist of the brain and the psychiatrist of the mind.

One of the greatest stimuli for reconsidering our approach to mental disorders in later life is the relative difficulty in recruitment that has been experienced, particularly in North America, in the fields of geriatric medicine and to some extent geriatric psychiatry. Martin's vision for the future largely ignores the field of geriatrics and instead focuses on the need for the convergence of psychiatry, neurology and neuroscience.

In 2005, Insel and Quirion made an impassioned plea for psychiatry to have an impact on public health by helping mental disorders to be understood and treated as brain disorders. This came from the heads of the respective national Mental Health Institutes in the United States and Canada at that time. In the past, mental disorders immediately became the purview of neurology the moment a lesion in the brain was identified. Like Martin, they note that development of more advanced neuroimaging techniques has helped to identify discrete structural and functional changes evident in many psychiatric disorders. What follows logically from their premise is that if mental disorders are indeed primarily brain disorders, then the fundamentals of psychiatry must of necessity include a greater emphasis on neuroscientific principles. Increased knowledge regarding the neuroscientific basis of psychiatry is already impacting clinical practice and the training of future psychiatrists. In tandem with this, a concern has been raised that if psychiatry becomes a neuroscience-based disorder, we may lose the discipline's sophisticated understanding of personality development and environmental or interpersonal contributions to human behaviour.

Insel and Quirion noted that advances in molecular genetics, identifying genetic and epigenetic variations in disease, have facilitated increased understanding of many mental disorders and in turn revealed new targets for treatment. There is now increased understanding regarding how environmental and biological factors can interact to precipitate psychiatric morbidity in vulnerable individuals. These findings sustain the idea that the future of psychiatry as a clinical neuroscience discipline is dependent upon successful incorporation of molecular genetics, neuroscience and psychosocial factors. Increased neuroscientific understanding should only serve to enhance therapeutic efficacy regardless of whether interventional strategies are considered to be primarily 'biological' or psycho-social in nature.

Neuroimaging research involving advanced structural, functional and molecular tech-niques may help with development of biomarkers for mental disorders. For example, recent research has started to characterise depressive biotypes according to patterns of activation and underactivation in distinct neural networks creating possibilities for more targeted treatment based upon neurobiology rather than symptomatic presentation, which often maps poorly onto underlying network dysfunction. Similarly, advances in pharmacogenet-ics now allow more targeted selection of pharmacological interventions based upon indi-vidual variations in drug metabolism and pharmacodynamic factors linked to treatment response. While many of these advances have yet to percolate through to routine clinical practice, increasing development and validation of biomarkers together with decreasing costs and increased availability of advanced neuroimaging and molecular technologies mean that these changes are likely to have an increasing impact upon clinical practice over time.

Future Training in Clinical Neuroscience

The notion of the clinical neuroscientist was developed originally by Thomas Detre and advanced by others, including Insel and Quirion. If the fundamental premise is that mental disorders, such as AD, late life depression, paranoid disorders of late life and delirium are indeed brain disorders, then psychiatrists of the future will need to become brain scientists. Neurologists will necessarily have to incorporate a greater understanding of psychosocial influences into their practice, while psychiatrists must incorporate a greater understanding of the neuroscientific basis of psychiatric 'disease'. Insel and Quirion argue that redefining psychiatry as a clinical neuroscience will accelerate the re-integration of psychiatry with the rest of medicine. In the context of POA, this will mean closer integration with the disciplines of neurology and geriatric medicine. The misguided thesis of Cartesian dualism, with separation of mental health and psychiatric care from other medical care in the latter part of the twentieth century, served to perpetuate the stigma associated with mental illness for patients, families and those involved in their care. In addition, the separation of mental healthcare from the mainstream of medicine has had an adverse impact upon the quality of care provided to those with serious mental illness. The success of this future integration will depend on the ability of psychiatry to bring a modern neuroscientific approach to the healthcare needs of those who experience mental illness while retaining a focus upon the contribution of human experience to brain disease.

The reciprocal relationship of neurology and psychiatry is reflected in mirror papers by two leading researchers in the psychiatry of old age. Jeffrey Cummings, writing in 2005 on the neuropsychiatric burden of neurologic diseases in the elderly, highlighted the increasing recognition that brain dysfunction is also reflected by behavioural and affective symptoms in addition to intellectual and functional decline. Therefore, the management of brain disorders requires the involvement of psychogeriatricians and psychogeriatric services in order to manage conditions where behavioural and psychological symptoms are common and significant yet under-recognised and under-treated.

In the same issue of *International Psychogeriatrics*, John O'Brien reviewed the cognitive effects of traditional 'psychiatric disorders' such as schizophrenia, depression and bipolar disorder. O'Brien notes that in the prototypic psychiatric disorder, schizophrenia, cognitive impairment has been demonstrated in several areas, including working memory, attention, verbal and visual learning and memory, problem-solving and speed of processing. Similarly, depressed subjects have shown multiple impairments in attention, working memory, visual and verbal memory as well executive dysfunction. These cognitive deficits are not only a result of the mood disturbance (state) but persist even after recovery from the mood disorder (trait). Depression in older adults often may be considered a neurocognitive disorder which necessarily requires not only a focus upon symptomatic remission of depression but also a focus upon underlying neurobiological abnormalities precipitating and perpetuating the behavioural disturbance.

It is critical that psychosocial contributions to psychiatric illness (and indeed to non-psychiatric illness) are not neglected and that care needs are addressed in a comprehensive approach integrating good psychosocial care with good general medicine and neuroscience. Neuroscientific advances have increased understanding regarding how psychotherapeutic interventions work at a neurobiological level, and ongoing research in this area aims to increase understanding regarding predictors of treatment response to facilitate more targeted treatment. A greater emphasis upon short-term evidenced-based, manualised therapies has ensured that psychotherapeutic interventions are now more accessible and can be delivered in a standardised way to a greater number of individuals. This has facilitated an increasing emphasis upon primary and secondary prevention. In addition, there is ongoing work regarding how to adapt the most effective components of psychotherapeutic interventions to older adults and examine novel approaches in those resistant to initial therapeutic approaches.

Age-Based versus Needs-Based Services: The Future of Geriatrics?

There is no doubt that the behemoth of neuroscience cannot be ignored in the future development of POA, particularly in terms of our understanding mental disorders and their treatment. However, clinical and service delivery issues will not be addressed adequately by the traditional approach of neurology or neuroscientists. For this, we must turn to the sister disciplines of old age psychiatry and geriatric medicine. In these subspecialties, debates in the United Kingdom reflected the tension between ongoing development of age-based (geriatric) services and disorder-based services. Central to this argument was the idea that services should be available based on need rather than age alone. Proponents of the argument were opposed to the automatic transfer of patients from younger adult to older adult services simply because they pass the age of 65. Indeed, some younger adults who have multiple physical comorbidities, cognitive impairment and frailty may be better served by older adult services. On the other hand, older adults who are otherwise physically fit and may have been known to adult services may best be served by the same adult service. However, older adults who present for the first time late in life with a major mental disorder are more likely to need old age specialist services. The point of developing needs-based services is to ensure that service developments in one sector of the healthcare system do not have unintended adverse consequences for individuals who use the service in a different sector. In order for this to happen, government and local health services require a comprehensive vision for the healthcare service.

The Faculty of Old Age Psychiatry in the United Kingdom countered that while the notion of age-inclusive services sounds equitable, one of the reasons why old age psychiatry was necessary as a discipline was that older adults were often excluded from general services.

In addition, the particular health needs of older adults were often overlooked in a service largely configured towards the provision of care for younger adults. They argued that the politically popular emphasis on 'choice' in future health services may not auger well for older adults. There was a concern that by emphasising 'choice' under the rubric of 'integration', older adults would only be given lip service in terms of access. Old age psychiatrists and geriatric specialty services need to be advocates for older adults. Some have argued that to counter the impact of 'choice' and the erosion of geriatrics, geriatricians should take a lead in delivering hospital-based services that are of particular relevance to older people. Others have argued that geriatrics should be redefined as the clinical management of multiple long-term conditions. Indeed, the management of chronic disease is a priority in most developed healthcare services. Putting the emphasis on long-term chronic conditions may be easier to accept than simply being 'geriatric'.

Summary

Health services around the world face the challenge of a growing population of older adults with a high prevalence of psychiatric and cognitive disorders. There is a growing consensus that clinical neurosciences must influence the future understanding and management of 'psychiatric' disorders in late life. However, the psychosocial perspective based in traditional psychiatry must be preserved both in terms of service delivery and instilling a holistic, humane and empathic approach to older adults, their families and caregivers. We hope that diversity in approaches to this challenge will yield evidence-based, practical solutions that improve the quality of care of older individuals and families struggling to cope with these disorders.

Further Reading

Articles

Cowan, W. M. and Kandel, E. R. (2001). Prospects for neurology and psychiatry. *JAMA*, 285, 594–600. doi: 10.1001/jama.285.5.594.

Thoughtful article about the future of these two disciplines.

Cummings, J. L. (2005). The neuropsychiatric burden of neurological diseases in the elderly. *International Psychogeriatrics*, 17, 341–351. doi:10.1017/s1041610205002206.

Article mentioned earlier in the chapter.

Drysdale, A. T. *et al.* (2017). Resting-state connectivity biomarkers define neurophysiological subtypes of depression. *Nature Medicine*, 23, 28–38. doi: 10.1038/nm.4246.

An example of how biomarker research may facilitate more targeted treatment selection in the future.

Geschwind, D. H. and Flint, J. (2015). Genetics and genomics of psychiatric disease. *Science*, 349, 1489–1494. doi: 10.1126/science. aaa8954.

An overview of how genetics and genomics can increase understanding for mechanisms in common neuropsychiatric disorders.

Insel, T. R. and Quirion, R. (2005). Psychiatry as a clinical neuroscience discipline. *JAMA*, 294, 2221–2223. doi:10.1001/jama .294.17.2221.

These authors argue that psychiatry's future is as a neuroscience discipline.

Kandel, E. R. (1998). A new intellectual framework for psychiatry. *American Journal of Psychiatry*, 155, 457–469. doi: 10.1176/ajp.155.4.457.

See comments earlier in the chapter.

Martin, J. (2002). The integration of neurology, psychiatry, and neuroscience in the 21st century. *American Journal of Psychiatry*, 159, 695–704. doi: 10.1176/appi.ajp.159.5.695.

This article argues for the integration of these disciplines.

O'Brien, J. (2005). Dementia associated with psychiatric disorders. *International Psychogeriatrics*, 17 (Suppl. 1), S207–S221. doi: 10.1017/S1041610205002036.

See earlier in the chapter.

Book

Lock, M. (2014). *The Alzheimer Conundrum: Entanglements of Dementia and Aging*. Princeton, NJ: Princeton University Press.

An anthropologist brings her skills to bear on old age psychiatry, highlighting three burning questions for the future.

Index

Printed in the United States
by Baker & Taylor Publisher Services